HISTORY AND PHYSICAL EXAMINATION WORKBOOK
A Common Sense Approach

Mark Kauffman, DO, PA
Director of Physical Diagnosis—Problem Based Pathway Program
Clinical Assistant Professor of Family Medicine
Lake Erie College of Osteopathic Medicine

Co-Medical Director—Physical Assistant Department
Gannon University,
Erie, PA

Michele M. Roth-Kauffman, JD, MPAS, PA-C
Chair of the Physician Assistant Department
Associate Dean—College of Sciences, Engineering, and Health Sciences
Gannon University,
Erie, PA

JONES AND BARTLETT PUBLISHERS
Sudbury, Massachusetts
BOSTON   TORONTO   LONDON   SINGAPORE

World Headquarters

Jones and Bartlett Publishers
40 Tall Pine Drive
Sudbury, MA 01776
978-443-5000
info@jbpub.com
www.jbpub.com

Jones and Bartlett Publishers
Canada
6339 Ormindale Way
Mississauga, Ontario
L5V 1J2
CANADA

Jones and Bartlett Publishers
International
Barb House, Barb Mews
London W6 7PA
UK

Jones and Bartlett's books and products are available through most bookstores and online booksellers. To contact Jones and Bartlett Publishers directly, call 800-832-0034, fax 978-443-8000, or visit our website www.jbpub.com.

Substantial discounts on bulk quantities of Jones and Bartlett's publications are available to corporations, professional associations, and other qualified organizations. For details and specific discount information, contact the special sales department at Jones and Bartlett via the above contact information or send an email to specialsales@jbpub.com.

Copyright © 2007 by Jones and Bartlett Publishers, LLC.
ISBN 13: 978-0-7637-4340-6
ISBN 10: 0-7637-4340-2

The author has made every effort to ensure the accuracy of the information herein. However, appropriate information sources should be consulted, especially for new or unfamiliar procedures. It is the responsibility of every practitioner to evaluate the appropriateness of a particular opinion in the context of actual clinical situations and with due considerations to new developments. The author(s) and publisher disclaim all responsibility for any liability, loss, injury, or damage incurred as a consequence, directly or indirectly, of the use and application of any of the contents of this volume.

6048

Production Credits
Executive Editor: David Cella
Production Director: Amy Rose
Production Assistant: Rachel Rossi
Editorial Assistant: Lisa Gordon
Associate Marketing Manager: Laura Kavigian
Manufacturing Buyer: Amy Bacus
Composition: Paw Print Media
Cover Design: Kristin E. Ohlin
Printing and Binding: Courier Stoughton
Cover Printing: Courier Stoughton

Printed in the United States of America
12 11 10 09 08   10 9 8 7 6 5 4 3 2

Dedication

We would like to dedicate this book to our twins, Adam and Kevin Kauffman. May you achieve everything you truly desire through hard work and love.

AUTHOR BIOGRAPHIES

Mark Kauffman graduated from Saint Francis College of Loretto, Pennsylvania with a BS Physician Assistant in 1990 and was a member of the surgical transplant team at Pittsburgh's Children's Hospital until 1996, when he returned to medical school. He received his Doctor of Osteopathy degree from Lake Erie College of Osteopathic Medicine in 2000. He received board certification in Family Practice in 2003 and now practices primary care at the Erie Veteran's Administration, in Erie, Pennsylvania. He is currently the Director of Physical Diagnosis for the Problem Based Pathway Program and Clinical Assistant Professor of Family Medicine at the Lake Erie College of Osteopathic Medicine, and is Co-Medical Director of the Physician Assistant Department at Gannon University, in Erie, Pennsylvania.

Michele M. Roth-Kauffman graduated from Saint Francis College of Loretto, Pennsylvania with a BS Physician Assistant in 1990 and worked in surgery at St. Francis Medical Center in Pittsburgh, Pennsylvania until 1997. She obtained her Juris Doctorate from Duquesne University in 1996, and her MPAS in 2002. She is currently Chair of the Physician Assistant Department at Gannon University, and Associate Dean of the College of Sciences, Engineering, and Health Sciences.

CONTENTS

INTRODUCTION

The best way to learn how to perform a complete history and physical examination is to incorporate both into the study of medicine from the very beginning of your schooling. The good news is that taking histories and performing physicals require no—that's right—NO memorization. True, at the beginning, some mnemonics may aid you in getting back on track when you've lost your way, but these are soon forgotten as your skills in logical thinking take over.

If there is one goal for this Workbook, it is to encourage your common sense, hence the title. Please do not memorize the "Flows," because you will encounter them so often in your daily routine that they will become standard procedure without effort. There are some classic memory aids such as, "On Old Olympus Towering Tops," for the cranial nerves, and you will undoubtedly invent some of your own. But when you resort to your logic, you are more apt to understand the material instead of memorizing it.

This clinical workbook is intended to quicken your orientation to performing history and physical examinations. This is probably one of the few times in your studies when you are told NOT to read ahead for certain sections. Chapter 1, *Interviewing as an Art*, is a light exploration of the thought processes and actions behind obtaining a history. This includes what one does prior to walking into a patient room that will lead to a more accurate patient history. Why is history so important? It has been said that 90 percent of diagnoses are made by the history alone. Thus, if you don't take a good a history, you may not arrive at the correct diagnosis.

Chapter 2 discusses the techniques involved with clinical history gathering. Chapter 3 begins the history flows and should not be read ahead of time. Each encounter is designed for you and a partner, who acts as your patient. Your patient is given the presentation, and you ask the questions to find out why he or she is seeing you. Early on, you will likely not get a diagnosis. But you should still guess, as this is the very essence of why we take histories. As your medical studies progress, your goal should be to walk away from the case with at least three possibilities, and be able to determine a differential diagnosis.

The next chapter brings you into the physical examination and approaches the body in a logical progression, essentially from head to toe. Read ahead for this class because you will be performing the examination on your partner "patient." The physical examination "Flows" in Chapter 4 are presented in the order in which I typically do them in my own practice. That does not mean that you will perform these exams in exactly the same order. In time, you will develop your own order.

After completing an abdominal exam, for example, I immediately feel for the femoral pulses, which in my mind lie right below the abdomen in the inguinal area. From there, I complete the rest of the peripheral vascular exam, and then switch over to the musculoskeletal system, examining the joints first. If you reach the bottom of the abdomen and it makes you logically think of the longest nerve in the body—the vagus—then do the neurological examination next. There is no right or wrong method, only completeness.

Both history and exam are brought together in Chapter 5, which covers the "Comprehensive Flow." Once again, do not read this chapter ahead. You will want to experience walking into the patient's room, asking why he or she is there, developing a differential diagnosis, and performing a problem-specific examination.

Finally, the logistics of order writing is detailed in Chapter 6.

It is at this point that I usually apologize to my students in advance. You see, I am becoming my father. Let me explain. Most of the interviews in this book are the same ones I have experienced with real patients. Some are funny, some are sad, and a few are distillations of many experiences into a single example, but all of them are real. I like to teach by telling stories. So, the benefit of having this text in a written form is that I won't be repeating the same stories over and over again, like my Dad always does. Unfortunately, those of you in my class will be subjected to the overexposure.

One last point: relax and have fun. Help each other. You will learn from your peers and your patients for the rest of your lives. Study hard, but if you can't laugh at yourself, you will miss out on much of the experience of being human.

True Story

Early in my career when I was doing an emergency medicine rotation in Rochester, New York, I was sitting in a crowded lunch lecture. The presentation was on emergency bleeds. A physician came in the room and remarked that the topic was appropriate because a patient had just arrived in the ER who had bleeding varices that were life threatening. To my credit, instead of raising my hand to comment, I quietly leaned over to my supervisor who was sitting next to me and asked how someone could bleed to death in the scrotum. She didn't even laugh. She explained that it was *esophageal varies*, not a *scrotal varicocele*. With chagrin, I embarked down the humble trail of my study of medicine.

INTERVIEWING AS AN ART

1

Gathering the history from a patient interview is not simply asking questions and receiving an answer. Interpretation of the patient's true complaint requires intuition and the skill to observe as much of what is not said as what is said.

True Story

A young undergraduate student of medicine visited the emergency room with the complaint of "abdominal pain." The nursing staff screened him and triaged his complaint for the physician. But when the physician came around the curtain and inquired about his pain, the patient promptly requested a specific medication for the treatment of pubic lice. He presented one of the little critters that he had harvested from himself and placed in a bag for easy identification. At least he hadn't shaved one half of his pubic hair and set the other side on fire!

In this case, the complaint of abdominal pain to the nurse was the student's "admission ticket" to save himself from embarrassment. When the physician arrived, he promptly disclosed the true reason for seeking medical attention. However, this is not always the case. A patient may discuss dizziness for 30 minutes and as you start to walk out of the door say, "Oh, by the way, can I get something to help me sleep?" Sleep deprivation was the true reason for the patient coming in for a visit, but he or she may have been afraid of appearing to be drug-seeking.

Other patients may not even know their true complaint. The "frequent flyer," that is, the patient who is in the office one week for muscle aches, the next for "funny heart beats," and two weeks later for constipation, may truly be suffering from depression. As the astute provider, you need to discern the underlying problem that the patients themselves do not recognize.

Mindset

What is the purpose of seeing a patient? The answer is to take care of the patient's complaint. Every note needs a *chief complaint* and we will return to this issue in more depth in Chapter 2. The patient's complaint may be as simple as needing a physical examination for a driver's license, a bloody nose, or wanting you to examine a mole that just doesn't look right. Or, it may be as complex as unexplained weight loss, dizziness, or fatigue.

In any case, your goals during the interview are to not only gather information, but also to gain the trust of the patient. Gaining trust allows you to gather information that the patient may not otherwise share.

True Story

A mom brought her 16-year-old daughter into the ER for a urinary tract infection. The symptoms were classic as her daughter was experiencing burning on urination, frequency, and lower abdominal pain. Interestingly, the patient never had a urinary tract infection before. Ordinarily, part of the history would include a sexual history. When I asked the patient if she was sexually active, her mom promptly laughed, joking, "she knows I'd kill her." The daughter laughed, too. I completed the examination and turned to the mom, explaining that her daughter was becoming a young lady and this was a chance to develop relationships and trust with physicians. I asked if I could just summarize the history with her daughter alone. The mom agreed and stepped out.

I then turned and told the young lady that there were several things that I was required by law to report: sexual or physical abuse, and the desire of the patient to hurt herself or others. Other than those things, anything she had to share with me would be strictly confidential unless she asked me to share the information with others. That said, I promptly described how common it was to develop urinary tract infections after first starting a sexual relationship. I explained that treatments could be greatly different if I thought I was treating a "regular old urinary tract infection" or if the infection may be related to a sexual relationship. I again asked if there was anything she might tell me that could help me treat her in the best way possible. Without hesitation, she confided that she and her boyfriend of 2 years just started having sex. What a great opportunity to go beyond diagnosis and treatment! Not only could I tell her about the treatment for a urinary tract infection, as the urine dip stick proved she had, but I also got to educate her about sexually transmitted disease prevention and pregnancy. And as an extra bonus, the warm smile I got as she left told me she was likely to be open with future providers as well.

Heading for the Room

Okay. Your mindset is in place and you're feeling ready to solve the mystery waiting for you in the examination room. You grab the doorknob and open the door. Hold on! The history and physical exam begin outside of the patient room. How far outside, do you ask? On more than one occasion I've watched patients from my window as they whipped into the parking lot, jumped out of the car, and run into the office because they were late for their appointment. But when I went into the room, that same patient couldn't get up off of the table for me to examine them because their back hurt so badly. Do you see something wrong with this picture?

Chart Review: On the Outside, Looking In

Typically, some sort of chart is available before you go into the room. In the emergency room, it may be as simple as a one-line complaint and the vital signs. In the family practice office, however, you may have years of history in your hands. Before entering the examination room, the provider should review the chart and become familiar with the patient's name, age, and gender. Chest pain in a 7-year-old girl varies greatly in possible etiologies than a 75-year-old man. Reviewing the chart before going in the door allows you to quickly gather data that will help you to prepare for the interview.

Factors to note include:

- Demographics: age, sex, race (Anemia in an African-American? Maybe it's sickle cell.)
- Problem List: prior diagnoses ("I see you've had urinary tract infections before.")
- Last Problem: how long ago and why ("Did that mole we checked last time change at all?")
- Medications: list of current and past medications ("You're feeling dizzy? Maybe it's your atenolol.")
- Chief Complaint: The reason why they are here today.

A word of caution: don't let yourself become biased before you see the patient. After being in practice awhile, it is very easy to look at the chief complaint and say, "Oh no. It's Jim again for his back pain at 4:30 on a Friday afternoon. I'll bet he's out of pain pills." Approach each patient as you would your own family members (at least, the ones you like). Do not allow a person's race, gender, sexual orientation, substance abuse, "frequent flyer" status, mental illness, or any other characteristic cloud your judgment.

True Story

A patient diagnosed with schizophrenia who was well known to doctors in our emergency department presented with back pain. It was common for her to appear in the ERs all over our city on the weekends when her primary care center was closed. On this particular Sunday, she had been very busy at the admitting desk, telling everyone she had already been to the two biggest hospitals in town. She had been seen and discharged with mild analgesics for her complaint of left-sided back pain. As tempting as it may have been to do a cursory exam and send her on her way, something about the story didn't fit her pattern. Yes, she was known to jump around from ER to ER, but not on the same weekend. A thorough exam revealed weakness in flexion of her left leg. Final diagnosis: She had a staghorn kidney stone that was so big, it had eroded through her left kidney and caused an abscess to form in the psoas muscle. The moral of this story is to always give someone the benefit of the doubt. Approach each patient like it is the first time you saw them.

Entering the Room

By now you have read through the available data about this patient and have already begun to form an idea of what his/her needs may be. While you are conveniently standing outside the door reading the chart, you hear Mr. Carabooz (there are too many Mr. Jones's) coughing his head off inside of the room. You've already got a good idea of what's going on with him, so you may want to grab a mask. Walking in, you address the patient appropriately:

> "Hello, Mr. Carabooz. I'm student doctor/physician assistant/nurse practitioner (my name). What can I do for you today?"

I always use proper titles if meeting someone for the first time, such as Mr. or Ms. Addressing the patient by name immediately focuses the encounter to a more personal level. You then can ask what they would prefer to be called. If you are unsure of the pronunciation of a last name, simply introduce yourself first and then ask the patient how to pronounce their name correctly. Notice the open-ended question, "What can I do for you today?" This is telling the patient that you want to hear his or her story. Other options could include, How are you today? What brings you in today? I'll be taking care of you today. How can I help?

Even with this simple introduction there can be some sticky situations. For example, some people do not shake hands. I was quite surprised the first time I offered my hand and it was refused. No, it wasn't from a germaphobe. It was the mother of a transplant patient whose particular religious beliefs led her to refrain from hand shaking. It is easy to feel insulted at first. But all cultures are different, and whether you agree with the practice or not, respect is due. How would you approach the more serious situation where a child who has undergone a bone marrow transplant (bone marrow, the "mother of all blood products") develops a severe anemia and needs a blood transfusion, but his parents refuse because it is against their religion? Their religion allows the child to receive a bone marrow transplant, but this patient could die because she or he is prohibited from receiving even a pint of blood. What's to be done? In my experience, I ask for literature about their beliefs so that I can understand their religious laws and respect them. That doesn't mean that I have to agree with their decisions, but at least I understand them better.

Some cultures do not allow a male to examine a female. It's pretty difficult to diagnose a skin disorder if you aren't allowed to see the skin. Again, this true story illustrates my point: Having cultural awareness heightens your ability to obtain a thorough history.

Establishing Rapport

Establishing rapport is essential for developing trust between the provider and patient. Once trust has developed, the patient is more apt to confide in the provider. "Yeah, that cholesterol probably went up because I've kind of been forgetting to take my medication." Rapport is established by being thorough and showing genuine interest in the patient. When the provider displays compassion, then the relationship moves beyond the mechanical problem/diagnosis routine. By being kind, friendly, and cheerful, and by displaying a sense of humor and a smile, the provider develops the kind of "bedside manner" that patients value.

Attitudes about providers include perceptions of personal appearance and nonverbal communication. Studies have shown that patients subconsciously relate the competence of a provider to the style of clothing she or he wears. A provider rounding on the weekend in jeans and sneakers is deemed less competent than someone who is rounding in scrubs and clogs, who actually may be more competent than the provider who rounds in a suit and tie, or dress.

Ideally, there will be a bond of mutual respect between physician/provider and patient. The provider must choose vocabulary suitable to the level of the patient's education. Phrase questions in simple language appropriate to the patient's level of understanding. "Have you been having any palpitations?" isn't a question that I would ask the majority of my patients. But, "Is your heart beating fast?" is more appropriate. Avoiding the use of medical jargon helps establish a sense of uncomplicated communication.

Nonverbal Communication

Communication between two people is usually one third nonverbal. The words spoken aloud often are affirmed or negated nonverbally with body posture, type and duration of eye contact, and tone of voice communicating one's personal attitudes and emotions. Nonverbal communications are not under conscious control, so the messages are more likely to be genuine.

Posture is an important factor in conveying an image of confidence and competence. Standing erect, moving briskly with head up and stomach in are characteristic of the confident provider. A listless or lethargic appearance may be interpreted as a lack of concern. The provider shows interest and concern by maintaining an attentive position, sitting forward in the chair with an attentive facial expression and the head slightly tilted.

I was astounded when an attending physician with whom I was doing a psychiatry rotation sat back in his chair and began to open letters and peruse his mail while the patient was telling him his problems. This is inexcusable. Our eyes are our principle organs of expression. We express sincerity and interest with our eyes. Frequent eye contact is a necessity for telling the patient nonverbally that we are engaged in the encounter. In this age of electronic records, this interaction can be challenging as our eyes are drawn to the screen. If I am meeting the patient for the first time, I apologize in advance for looking at the screen:

> "I'm sorry, Mrs. Clark. We have electronic medical records so I may be looking
> at the computer screen a lot, but I promise that I am listening."

In the United States, a handshake is the most socially acceptable method of introduction. Again, be considerate of cultural differences where handshakes are not customarily used. Touching can be an effective method for communicating concern or compassion, and can break down some defensive barriers to communication. A general rule of thumb is to keep contact brief and limited to the lower arm. After establishing rapport, there is nothing unacceptable about sharing a hug with your patient who is distressed over the loss of her husband.

NOTES:

HISTORY TAKING

2

Without exception, each encounter MUST begin with the *chief complaint*. This is the reason the patient came in to see you. It is often documented in the patient's own words. The statement should be concise and describe the symptoms, diagnosis, or other reasons for the encounter. The following are several examples of how chief complaints should be documented:

"I have a urinary tract infection."

Follow-up congestive heart failure.

"My toe hurts."

Let's use, "I have a urinary tract infection" as the chief complaint. This is why the patient is in your office, and it is explained in her own words. Now, as you may remember from Chapter 1, Miss Smith may not actually have a urinary tract infection, but in her opinion, it is why she's there to see you.

The chief complaint may also include duration of time. I highly recommend gleaning out this information as it may change the possible etiologies of the complaint significantly.

"I have chest pain" × 3 hours.

"I have chest pain" × 23 years.

You may laugh, but I saw the second guy in the ER just the other day. The sense of urgency with the patient reporting 3 hours of chest pain varies greatly from that in the gentleman with 23 years of chest pain, who said he just wanted another opinion.

History of Present Illness (HPI)

The history of present illness (HPI) is the subjective story given to you by the patient in response to the questions you pose. Think "subjective" because it is subject to change.

True Story

While in the ER as a resident, I went to interview an 80 something year-old female who was being evaluated for chest pain. During the interview, I found that her pain had actually occurred twice. The first time happened after she had dropped a pencil under her kitchen table. She said that as she stretched out her arm trying to get it, she felt a sharp pull across the front of her chest that lasted only for a few seconds. The second time occurred as she lifted up her garbage can to take it out to the curb for the garbage collectors. Again, she had experienced the same sharp pull across her chest. I asked a host of other questions, all of which led to my diagnosis of a musculoskeletal origin of her chest pain. Confidently, I went back and presented this elderly patient's case to my attending physician, urging a short course of mild analgesics. After my presentation, the attending re-interviewed my patient. Her subsequent description was of a squeezing, crushing, left-sided chest pain that had occurred only after dragging the garbage can down 50 yards of driveway. The patient was admitted to rule out a myocardial infarction.

This story illustrates that the patient's history is subject to change. We will talk about the objective physical examination in Chapter 4.

Opening Question

One of the keys to obtaining an accurate history is to allow your patient to tell you their story first. The first question should be open-ended like the examples above. *Open-ended* simply means that the question cannot be answered with a "yes" or "no" response. It requires further explanation. Asking, "What brings you in today?" forces the patient to begin telling you a story. If his or her response fails to give you details (i.e., "I have chest pain"), then the original question is followed by another open-ended question or statement (i.e., "Oh, tell me about that.")

However, some patients do need to be directed. "Well, the first time I had chest pain was back in 1962, when I was visiting my sister Gwendolyn in Florida. Lovely place she has really. Her house was built back in the 1920s. Once she found an original painting by..." You get the idea. If you didn't redirect this patient, you would need to have pizza sent in for dinner. A response to this type of stream of consciousness can be, "I'm sorry to interrupt, and if we have time, we can come back to that, but can you tell me when you had the chest pain last?" It may take several redirections in a case like this to keep the information on track. Notice that this second question became more specific.

If a patient is unable to answer an open-ended question, you may then move on to close-ended questions, those that require a yes/no or more specific response. For example:

Open-ended: "Describe the chest pain."

"I don't know, it just hurts."

Close-ended: "Is it sharp, dull, achy, pressure, squeezing?"

Logical Sequence

Again, my primary goal with this text is to help you to think logically. I do not want you to memorize anything. One answer from the patient often leads to the next question. Your role is to keep the patient on track with exploring his or her chief complaint while also gaining sufficient information to obtain an accurate diagnosis. There are several thought processes behind your questions.

	Question	Thought Process
Provider:	"Do you drink alcohol?"	Social history screening question
Patient:	"Yes."	Positive screen
Provider:	"How often do you drink?"	Follow-up question to positive screen
Patient:	"Every day."	Oh my, that's a lot.
Provider:	"How much do you drink in a day?"	Quantifier
Patient:	"Oh, only one glass of wine a day."	Well that's good for the heart.

Do you see how the picture changes? You go from thinking the person may be an alcoholic to recognizing the cardiovascular benefits of moderate alcohol consumption. Now, if you had discovered that the patient had been in rehab six times over the last two years for alcohol abuse, you would immediately return to your original opinion that drinking on a daily basis is way too much.

Never leave a question with an incomplete answer open. If someone admits that they've had the same abdominal pain twice in the past, ask about those past occurrences. When were they? How long did they last? How did they get better?

Components of the History of Present Illness

In the past, I have presented the components of the HPI without any sequence. Why? It's because answers don't come from patients in any particular sequence. The fact that there is no standard list of questions does not mean that the questions are not in a logical order, however. For example, when a patient presents with dizziness, one of the first questions I ask is, "Describe what you mean by dizziness?" There are many other options to this line of questioning: "When did you first have this dizziness? Have you ever had this before?"

However, my students said that they needed something in the beginning that would get them back on tract if they got lost. They offered a mnemonic ("CODIERSMASH"), which I have modified to "CODIERSMMASSH" (Table 2-1). This mnemonic (which students say "rocks") helps the beginner student to take histories. I've even been known to mutter "CODIERSMMASSH" during practical examinations to corral the student back in line. The results have been amazing (and that's all the help they get!).

Certainly, anyone can get lost in asking questions to determine the patient's chief complaint and subsequent history. When you first take histories on real patients, you probably will have to return to the room several times to ask the questions you forgot the first time around.

Table 2-1   CODIERSMMASSH

Mnemonic	Overview	Specific Questions
C - Chronology	Time frame showing the sequence of events	Have you ever had this BEFORE? How has it CHANGED? What was the order of symptoms?
O - Onset	Occurrence	When did current symptoms start?
D - Description Duration	Describe it Length of time	What does it FEEL like? How LONG does it last?
I - Intensity	Scale	On a scale from 1 to 10, how bad is the pain?
E - Exacerbating factors		What makes it worse?
R - Remitting factors		What makes it better?
S - Symptoms associated	Concurrent findings	For a cold: Do you have a fever, chills?
M - Medications		Name, dose, frequency?
M - Medical history		Previous medical diagnoses?
A - Allergies		Food, environmental, drug – what happens?
S - Surgical history		What? When?
S - Social history		Tobacco, ETOH, drugs, education, occupation?
H - Hospitalization		What? Where? When?

Abbreviation: ETOH, alcohol abuse and related problems.

Not all histories will have every component of CODIERSMMASSH. For example, if someone is complaining of dizziness, you may be able to assign an imprecise intensity such as being so dizzy the patient fell down, or so dizzy that the patient couldn't go to work that day, so you may not use the "I" (intensity) at all. Some complaints lend themselves naturally to classic scales. A typical pain scale will span from 1 to 10, with 10 being the worst pain. Other complaints will have 12 associated symptoms. One example is someone complaining of shortness of breath, where you have to rule out a myocardial infarction, pneumonia, congestive heart failure, or deconditioning. Other histories may need only a few questions, such as the patient complaining about a brown spot on the arm.

Review of Symptoms (ROS)

The review of symptoms (ROS) is an inventory of symptoms related to the body's systems. It is documented separately from "CODIERSMMASSH." However, pertinent positive and negative components of the ROS are drawn up into the HPI and these mostly answer the question of "symptoms associated."

For example, if someone presents complaining of shortness of breath, the HPI would include components found in the ROS that help to rule in or rule out certain disease processes. To rule out pneumonia, you need to ask the patient about fever, chills, cough, and sputum production. To rule out congestive heart failure, you must ask about difficulty breathing while lying flat (orthopnea), sudden shortness of breath while sleeping (paroxysmal nocturnal dyspnea), dyspnea on exertion, and peripheral edema. The answers to these questions would be documented within the HPI.

It is important to recognize that the ROS is still part of the history, that is, the questions you ask and the answers you receive, and it is not the physical portion of the examination. Beginning students frequently document physical findings under the ROS, but this is a mistake. Table 2-2 contains several examples of ROS for each body area but is far from complete.

Table 2-2   Review of Symptoms (ROS)

System	Symptoms
Constitution	Fever, chills, weight loss or gain, night sweats, fatigue
Eyes	Blurred or loss of vision, double vision, eye pain, injection, discharge, deviation
Ears, nose, mouth, and throat	Ear pain, discharge, hearing loss, epistaxis, nasal congestion, lesions, tooth pain, dysphagia, tinnitus, sore throat
Cardiovascular	Palpitations, chest pain, peripheral edema, claudication, irregular heart beats, murmur
Respiratory	Shortness of breath, orthopnea, dyspnea on exertion, coughing, wheezing, chest pain, paroxysmal nocturnal dyspnea, hemoptysis
Gastrointestinal	Dyspepsia, nausea, vomiting, diarrhea, constipation, eructation, bloating, hematemesis, hematochezia, abdominal pain, change in caliber of the stools, bright red blood per rectum, melena
Genitourinary	Hesitancy, flank pain, dysuria, hematuria, urgency, frequency, decrease in force of stream, vaginal or penile discharge, dyspareunia, hematospermia
Musculoskeletal	Arthralgia, myalgia, boney deformity, weakness
Integumentary/breast	Changes in pigmentation or texture, rashes, lesions, pruritus, hair loss or change in hair texture, nail changes, dimpling
Neurologic	Facial asymmetry, memory loss, paresthesias, weakness, slurred speech, imbalance, changes in gait, dysphagia
Psychiatric	Depression, suicidal or homicidal ideation, anxiety, hallucinations
Endocrine	Polyuria, polyphagia, polydipsia, heat or cold intolerances
Hematologic/lymphatic	Easy bruising or bleeding, anemia, transfusion history, syncope, lymphadenopathy
Allergic/immunologic	Allergies, recurrent infections

Table 2-3 is a history taking worksheet. You may photocopy it for repeated use.

Table 2-3   Worksheet for History Taking

History Taking Worksheet   Patient: _____

CC: _____

HPI: _____

_____

_____

_____

_____

Medications:	Name	Dosage	Frequency	Name	Dosage	Frequency
	_____	_____	_____	_____	_____	_____
	_____	_____	_____	_____	_____	_____

Allergies with   Food _____

Reactions: Medications _____

                  Environmental _____

Hospitalizations:	Reason	Date	Surgeries:	Procedure	Date
	_____	_____		_____	_____
	_____	_____		_____	_____

Immunizations: Last: Td _____   Pneumonia _____   Influenza _____

Social History: Caffeine _____   Education _____
                  Tobacco _____   Occupation _____
                  Alcohol _____   Lives with _____
                  Drugs _____   Travel _____
                  Exercise _____   Diet _____
                  Age _____   Cause or medical condition _____

Family History: Mother   L/D _____
                  Father   L/D _____
                  Brothers L/D _____
                  Sisters   L/D _____

ROS: General   _____
Head   _____
Eyes   _____
Ears   _____
Nose   _____
Mouth   _____
Neck   _____
Respiratory   _____
Cardiac   _____
Gastrointestinal _____
Genitourinary   _____
Breast   _____
Musculoskeletal   _____
Neurologic   _____
Endocrine   _____
Psychiatric   _____

                                          Signature: _____

Abbreviations: CC, chief complaint; HPI, history of present illness; Td, tetanus and diphtheria toxoids; L/D, living/dead.

NOTES:

THE HISTORY FLOWS

3

This chapter presents clinical cases that are designed as partnered exercises in obtaining histories and should NOT be read in advance. Each partner is assigned to a role as either the provider or the patient. The patient reads the flow prior to the case in order to become familiar with the answers, which will allow for a smoother presentation. When the patient is ready, the provider begins the case with an introduction, including their name and title, an explanation as to their role, and an open-ended introductory question.

> "Hello, Mrs. Humphry, I am Student Doctor Stuart. I'll be taking your history and performing a short exam, and then we'll have Dr. Carrol come in. How can I help you?"

This clearly provides the patient with your name and level of education. The patient is aware of your role, and it reassures the patient that, as a student, you will not be making management decisions on your own, but will be discussing the patient with an advanced provider. The open-ended question that follows will allow the patient to begin their story with their chief complaint. The provider is then ready to elicit the HPI and all of its CODIERSMMASSH components (see Chapter 2).

At the beginning of your medical career, it is likely that you will focus on trying not to miss any of the questions that you believe need to be asked. As you no longer have to fall back on the mnemonic, you will begin to THINK instead of remember. You major goal is to develop a *differential diagnosis*, which is a list of possible etiologies for the patient's complaints, arranged in an order with the most likely diagnosis being presented first. As you become adept at taking histories, you will begin to formulate the diagnoses even before seeing the patient.

Standing outside the examination room, you hear the patient sneeze. Your differential diagnosis begins to form immediately: cold, environmental allergies. You open the chart and see that your patient is a 32-year-old female who was last seen for back pain that was diagnosed as a lumbar strain 6 months earlier. Her problem list shows that she is a smoker and that her only medication is birth control pills. The diagnoses expand: back pain, medication refill. Now you read the chief complaint as documented by the nurse: cough. This may add bronchitis to your list of diagnoses and yet you haven't seen the patient. What if she has chest pain and shortness of breath? Could she be having a pulmonary embolism? Her risk is increased because she is a smoker and on birth control pills.

This example demonstrates the constantly fluctuating possibilities of diagnoses. When you start the interview, your questions will either rule in or rule out each possible diagnosis. No shortness of breath or chest pain? She's likely not having a pulmonary embolism. She has a runny nose, itchy, watery eyes, and a tickle in the throat? Allergic rhinitis moves up on the list.

Flow Orientation

You should do one case as the provider and then switch roles with your partner and do another case as the patient. There is no "right" order to the questions, only one question leading to the next. Your practice exercises should be done as follows:

1. Pick the History Flow and allow the "patient" to review the answers.
2. When the patient is ready, the provider introduces him/herself and begins collecting the data for the HPI.
3. When the provider asks a question, the patient provides the answer and checks it off of the history flow.
4. When the provider has no further questions, the flow has been completed.
5. The provider should write up the case as shown in Table 2-1 or in Appendix A.
6. On the write-up, the provider should list three possibilities in the differential diagnosis.

As you first begin taking histories, you will be learning simply how to take a history and not the intricacies of medicine. Thus, your "symptoms associated" category is likely to be short. Your task will be to develop a logical sequence to your interviews. Concentrate on the time frame. What symptom developed first, had it ever occurred before, and how has it changed? Never let a question be answered incompletely.

"Describe the pain."

"It just hurts."

This does not answer the question. You are no further ahead in finding the cause of the pain than you were before you asked the question.

As your history taking skills and the depth of your medical knowledge increase, you will be able to intricately weave the components of the HPI together. When a 23-year-old woman presents with right knee pain, undoubtedly you will not take a sexual history. Why would you? Later, however, you will recognize that her knee pain may be caused by gonorrhea. This is a definite **Board question (BQ)**. Write it down.

Also, when first starting these Flows, you should not strictly limit your time. As you advance your skills, you should begin to limit each encounter to 7 minutes. This mimics a true patient encounter, which typically is a 15-minute appointment. You have 15 minutes to take your history, perform your problem-specific exam, and complete an assessment and plan while educating your patient and involving them in their own treatment. It does sound daunting, doesn't it?

The first case is followed by a sample write-up. You should practice writing up each case. Notice in the example that pertinent positives and negatives are grouped together. The time frame should be developed using a logical flow. If one question should have led to another, the follow-up question will be inset.

Provider's Question	Patient's Answer
"Do you smoke?"	"Yes."
"How much a day?"	"About a pack and a half."

All of these Flows are from actual encounters or a distillation of many examinations into a single example. The answers are those that came from real patients. Often they are not grammatically correct; they may demonstrate a misunderstanding by the patient or may even be offensive. These are aspects of patient care that providers encounter in regular practice and you must be able to efficiently handle these and other situations.

Following each Flow, the main clues will be discussed. Not every case has a pure diagnosis. There are many more questions that could have been asked for each case, but an attempt has been made to limit them to those of highest yield, while trying to keep the Flows to one page. If a question is asked that does not have an answer, the patient should reflect that they do not know or provide a simple answer. The Flows progressively become more clinically advanced.

Sample write-ups are shown in Appendix A. At this point, your write-up will contain only the subjective section and the assessment and plan, as you will not be doing a physical examination. The "subjective" section of a progress note or office visit correlates to the "HPI" in a complete history and physical exam. The assessment and plan can be grouped together for clarity, showing which intervention goes with what diagnosis. Abbreviations are found in Appendix B.

FED TACOS
GOOD EXERCISE   DRUGS   OCCUPATN
DRUGS   Alcohol   SEXUAL HX
CAFFEINE

CASE 1
16 y/o female c/o ear pain

LMP

Chief Complaint (CC): ear pain (antibiotics)

C - Chronology: ella winter (has it changed)

O - Onset: 3 days ago

D - Description: constant

Duration: 3 days

I - Intensity: 5

E - Exacerbating Factors: ~~Antihistimes~~ NO

R - Remitting Factors: Antihistamine

S - Symptoms Associated: drainage (yellow/green) clear nasal drainage
nothing

M - Medications: NO

M - Medical History: tubes in ears when younger, NKD Medical issues

A - Allergies: None

S - Surgical: tubes in ears.

S - Social Hx: F-Sine, Reg. Exercise, NOETOH, Smoke 1-2/day for 3 years, no drugs
Student (EtOH Sex Hx)

H - Hospitalization Hx: NO

1st day of last Period = 1 week ago

List three things in the Differential Diagnosis

OM/TS

Sinusitis

Allergies

think of Referred Pain

CASE 1
Write-Up

Date: _____

Time: _____

Chief Complaint: _____

_____

Subjective: _____

_____

_____

_____

_____

Assessment: _____

_____

_____

_____

_____

Plan: _____

_____

_____

_____

_____

Legible Signature: _____

CASE 1
16 y/o female c/o ear pain

_____ Introduces self and explains role.
_____ What brings you in today?   My ear hurts.

Chronology/Onset

_____ **When** did it start?   About 3 days ago.
_____ Did you ever have this **before**?   Yes.
_____ **When** was that?   It seems like every winter.
_____ **How** were you treated?   They gave me an antibiotic.
_____ Has it **changed** at all?   It was worse, but there felt like this sudden release of pressure.

Description/Duration

_____ Which **ear** is it?   My right one.
_____ Can you **describe** the pain?   It's an ache.

Intensity

_____ How bad is it on a **scale** from 1 to 10?   I'd say a 5.

Exacerbation

_____ What makes it **worse**?   Nothing really.

Remission

_____ What makes it **better**?   Antihistamines seem to help a little.

Symptoms associated

_____ Is there any **drainage**? ⌇ from ear   Yes, there is.
_____ What **color is it**? ⌇   Yellow or green, and it smells funny.
_____ Do you have a **stuffy/runny nose**?   Yes.
_____ What **color** is it?   It's just clear.
_____ Any **fever or chills**?   No.
_____ **Sore throat**?   No.
_____ **Hearing loss** or **dizziness**?   No.
_____ **Toothache**?   No.
_____ Surgical History?   I had tubes in my ears when I younger.

MMASSH

_____ Do you have any **medical** conditions?   No.
_____ Are you on any **medications**?   No.
_____ Do you have any **allergies**?   No.
_____ Do you **smoke**?   Yes.
_____ **How much a day**?   One or two cigarettes.
_____ **How long** have you been smoking?   Three years.
_____ When was the **FDLNMP**?   About a week ago.

Case Review #1: 16 y/o female c/o ear pain

In this case, we have a 16-year-old female. Although more commonly found in younger children, any age group can develop middle ear infections—otitis media—especially if they have a prior history of the same condition. It is also an age where adolescents frequently go swimming or use hot tubs, which leads one to think of an external ear infection, otitis externa.

These diagnoses are from the chief complaint only. She does have a prior history of ear pain that occurs mostly in the winter, which lessens the likelihood of an external ear infection and increases the likelihood of a middle ear infection because this is more common in the winter seasons. The key to diagnosis is the description by the patient of the sudden release of pain, likely the tympanic membrane rupturing, which correlates with the discharge from the ear that seems to be bacterial from the color and odor characteristics.

Questions to determine the other symptoms associated are in regard to what organs are likely to be affected also; these would include the nose and throat as well as fever and chills as signs of infection. MMASSH adds little to our diagnosis except that the patient may be more prone to infection as she is a smoker. Lastly, all women should be asked when the First Day of Last Normal Menstrual Period (FDLNMP) occurred, as you are likely going to be giving this patient an antibiotic and would not want to harm a fetus (see Table 3-1).

Note: Although both "FDLMP" (first day of last menstrual period) and "LMP" (last menstrual period) are often used as acronyms, there is a recent advancement toward a more precise delineation of the *exact* date. This is why we exclusively use the longer but more categorical "FDLNMP" acronym.

Table 3-1   Sample SOAP Note

Mnemonic	Description
CC (Chief Complaint):	Ear pain × 3 days
S (subjective):	16 y/o AA female presents with right ear pain × 3 days. She describes the pain as an ache, which had been of greater intensity, but is now at a level of 5/10 following a sudden release of pressure. Nothing has made the pain worse, and antihistamines have helped somewhat. She has had similar pain in the past, occurring mostly in the winter months. She admits to a yellow or green malodorous drainage from the right ear and nasal congestion with clear exudate. She denies fever, chills, or sore throat.
PMHX:	None
Medications:	Benadryl
Allergies:	None
Social Hx:	Smokes 1 to 2 cigarettes a day × 3 years
FDLNMP:	One week ago
O (objective):	The physical exam (PE) would follow here. You will learn documentation of the PE in Chapter 4.
A (Assessment):	List three things in the differential diagnosis for practice:
	Right otitis media
	Right otitis externa
	Upper respiratory tract infection
P (Plan):	To put in extra effort, decide how you would treat the diagnosis.
	Right otitis media: amoxicillin 250 mg qid × 10 days
	Increase fluids. Return to school in 2 days.
	Return to clinic in 2 weeks for recheck. Call earlier with no improvement, increase in pain, fever, or discharge.

CASE 2
12 y/o male with a rash

Presents with his mother who is answering most of the questions

Chief Complaint (**CC**): _____

C - Chronology: _____

O - Onset: _____

D - Description: _____

    Duration: _____

I - Intensity: _____

E - Exacerbating Factors: _____

R - Remitting Factors: _____

S - Symptoms Associated: _____

M - Medications: _____

M - Medical History: _____

A - Allergies: _____

S - Surgical: _____

S - Social Hx: _____

H - Hospitalization Hx: _____

List three things in the Differential Diagnosis

_____

_____

_____

CASE 2
Write-Up

Date: _____

Time: _____

Chief Complaint: _____

_____

Subjective: _____

_____

_____

_____

_____

_____

Assessment: _____

_____

_____

_____

_____

Plan: _____

_____

_____

_____

_____

Legible Signature: _____

CASE 2
12 y/o male with a rash

Presents with his mother who is answering most of the questions

_____ Introduces self and explains role.
_____ What brings you in today?   I have a rash.

Chronology

_____ Ever **had it before**?   I think, maybe last summer.
    _____ How did you treat it?   It just went away.
_____ Has it **changed** in appearance?   No, it just seems to be spreading.

Onset

_____ **When** did you first notice it?   A couple of days ago.

Description/Duration

_____ **Where** is it **(location)**?   All over.
    _____ Where did you **get it first**?   I think it started on my legs.
    _____ Then where did it go?   Then my belly and arms.

Exacerbation

_____ Does anything make it **worse**?   The heat makes it itch more.

Remission

_____ Does anything make it **better**?   A bath helped a little.

Symptoms associated

_____ Does it **itch**?   Yes.
_____ Do you have a **sore throat**?   No.
_____ Have you had a **fever**?   No.

Social History

_____ Did you have any **exposures** to anything?   I don't know.
_____ Were you out in the **woods or weeds** at all?   Probably.
_____ Any **new** laundry **detergents or deodorants**?   I don't do laundry (mom says no).
_____ Does anyone else you know have the same thing?   No.
_____ Have you been **bitten by anything**?   I don't think so.

MMASSH

_____ Any **Previous Medical Conditions**?   He has ADD.
_____ Are you on any **MEDICATIONS**?   He just started taking Ritalin.
    _____ When?   A couple of days ago.
_____ Were you ever **on it before**?   No.
_____ Do have any **ALLERGIES**?   No.
_____ Have you had any **SURGERIES**?   No.
_____ Any **hospitalizations**?   No.

Case Review #2: 12 y/o male with a rash

Many times you will be attempting to interview a patient but others in the room will be answering the questions, such as in this case. When evaluating an adolescent, I direct my questions and keep as much eye contact with the patient as possible, although parents often like to answer for them.

This seems like a fairly straightforward case. The patient developed a rash over the last several days. Location is important. Asking the patient where it started and the pattern of spread can help to differentiate the cause of the rash. For example, the rash associated with Rocky Mountain Spotted Fever (RMSF) usually starts on the wrists and ankles, and then spreads to the extremities and onto the trunk. The palms and soles are affected in RMSF but spared in other diseases. The character of pruritus suggests a possible contact dermatitis, prompting questioning of new detergents, outdoor activities, or other exposures. The fact that he had it last summer increases the likelihood of Rhus dermatitis (poison ivy or poison oak), but we would have been even more suspicious if his social history revealed that he had been camping in the last week. This case demonstrates the importance of completeness. In a 12-year old, you may discount his past medical history, but here, finding out that he has ADD and was just started on a new medication, allows you to add "drug reaction" to the differential diagnosis.

Your differential diagnosis may include:

1. Contact dermatitis
2. Drug reaction
3. Viral exanthema

Please note that you cannot use "rule out" as a primary diagnosis. For example, for the patient who comes in with chest pain, you cannot give the primary diagnosis:

Impression/Plan: Rule out myocardial infarction.

You can, however, write:

Impression/Plan: Chest pain r/o myocardial infarction.

CASE 3
23 y/o female complaining of a red eye

Chief Complaint (**CC**): _____

C - Chronology: _____

O - Onset:_____

D - Description: _____

　　　　Duration: _____

I - Intensity: _____

E - Exacerbating Factors: _____

R - Remitting Factors: _____

S - Symptoms Associated: _____

M - Medications: _____

M - Medical History: _____

A - Allergies: _____

S - Surgical: _____

S - Social Hx: _____

H - Hospitalization Hx: _____

List three things in the Differential Diagnosis

_____

_____

_____

CASE 3
Write-Up

Date: _____

Time: _____

Chief Complaint: _____

_____

Subjective: _____

_____

_____

_____

_____

_____

Assessment: _____

_____

_____

_____

_____

Plan: _____

_____

_____

_____

_____

Legible Signature: _____

CASE 3
23 y/o female complaining of a red eye

_____ Introduces self and explains role.	
_____ What brings you in today?	My eye is red.

Chronology/Onset

_____ **When** did it start?	Yesterday.
_____ What were you **doing**?	I just noticed it in the bathroom mirror.
_____ Did you ever have this **before**?	No.
_____ Has it **changed** at all?	It's redder today.

Description/Duration

_____ Which **eye** is it?	My left one.

Exacerbation

_____ Does anything make it **worse**?	No.

Remission

_____ What makes it **better**?	A warm washcloth helps a little.

Symptoms associated

_____ Is there any **pain**?	No.
_____ Do you have any **photophobia**?	No.
_____ Is there any **drainage/matting**?	Yes, there is.
_____ What **color is it**?	Yellow.
_____ Any **visual changes**?	It's a little blurry until I get the goop out.
_____ **Runny nose/sore throat**?	No.
_____ Does it **itch**?	Yes, it does.

MMASSH

_____ Do you have any **medical** conditions?	I am diabetic.
_____ Are you on any **medications**?	Metformin.
_____ Do you have any **allergies**?	No.
_____ Do you **smoke**?	Yes.
_____ **How much a day**?	Half a pack a day.
_____ **How long** have you smoked?	About 5 years.
_____ What is your **occupation**?	I work at a daycare center.
_____ **Contact with others** with the same?	Some of the kids have it, too.
_____ Do you wear **contact lenses**?	No.
_____ When was the **FDLNMP**?	About a week ago.

Case Review #3: 23 y/o female complaining of a red eye

When someone presents with a red eye, the diagnoses of viral and bacterial conjunctivitis immediately come to mind. Trauma is also a concern, which is quickly reviewed by asking a single question, and the method of discovery by the patient, solved by her statement that she simply looked into the mirror and saw that her eye was red.

One of the commonly missed questions in this Flow is, "Which eye?" The reason is quite simple. When a patient presents to you in a real setting and complains of a red eye, it is quite easy for us to identify which eye by looking at the patient. The red eye jumps out at us. At first I thought this was a minor point to include with this case, but then I was reminded that "wrong site surgery" is a leading reason of medical errors. "Tragic" does not fully describe the young basketball player who was diagnosed with bone cancer and awoke from the surgery to find that the surgeon had removed the wrong leg. It is better to practice clarifying which side the complaint is on now, ingraining the habit into your subconsciousness.

Matting and drainage correlate with conjunctivitis. The lack of photophobia and pain help to rule out acute glaucoma. This case demonstrates another incomplete answer. When you get a positive answer for drainage, you cannot stop. You must ask about the color of the drainage. Viral conjunctivitis may be clear and stringy, whereas bacterial conjunctivitis is often purulent.

Also important in patients who present with eye complaints is documenting the level of vision before your treatment is begun. Once we study the physical exam component (Chapter 4), you will be able to document acuity. Documenting diminished visual acuity prior to treatment clarifies that the loss was not a result of delayed or improper therapy.

Again, this case demonstrates the need for completeness. By eliciting the social history with regard to occupation, we help to rule out trauma (that might occur more frequently, e.g., in someone who is a machinist) and other exposures (e.g., daycare workers where conjunctivitis is notorious). After finding out this patient works in a daycare setting, it is important to ask if she has had any contact with others who have the same complaint or symptoms. This thought process also holds true for other infectious exposures. This is where we ask about other members of the family who may be experiencing the same symptoms, recent visits to hospitals or nursing homes, coworkers with symptoms, and the like.

FED TACOS w/back
its more importans
to know the
type of pain severity
intensity
(if anything
changes)

LIZ

CASE 4
26 y/o female c/o back pain

Chief Complaint (CC): _back pain_

C - Chronology: _lifting stack of anatomy textbooks_

O - Onset: _last night @ around midnight_

D - Description: _lower back (5 on scale of 1-10) burning, yup/led usisue)_
- Radiates into your right leg (hurt)

Duration: _pretty constant_

I - Intensity: _5_

E - Exacerbating Factors: _bending over or twisting the wrong way (hurt)_

R - Remitting Factors: _no movement (2 tabs of ibuprofin, 2+ hrs usually)_

S - Symptoms Associated: _no numbness or tingling, just pain, no weakness_

M - Medications: _depressed ibuprofen_

M - Medical History: _no other med hx_

A - Allergies: _allergic to bee stings_

S - Surgical: _tonsils removed (couple years ago)_

S - Social Hx: _coffee intake (2 cups of coffee a day)_

H - Hospitalization Hx: _none besides surgery_ last pd 1 week ago not sexually active

bowel frequency

List three things in the Differential Diagnosis

pinching of the nerve
pulled muscle (musuloskeletal)
pregnancy (ectopic)
menstrual
pinched nerve
kidneys → pain, fever, blood in urine, chills, brownish, smell

CASE 4
Write-Up

Date: _____

Time: _____

Chief Complaint: _____

_____

Subjective: _____

_____

_____

_____

_____

_____

Assessment: _____

_____

_____

_____

_____

Plan: _____

_____

_____

_____

_____

Legible Signature: _____

CASE 4
26 y/o female c/o back pain

_____ Introduces self and explains role.	
_____ What brings you in today?	I hurt my back.

Chronology/Onset

_____ Is it continuous or does it come and go?	It's continuous.
_____ **When** did you hurt it?	Last night at midnight.
_____ What were you **doing** at the time?	Lifting a stack of anatomy textbooks.
_____ How has it **changed**?	It hasn't really.
_____ Did you ever have this **before**?	No.

Description/Duration

_____ **Describe** the pain.	It feels like a pulled muscle, kind of like burning.
_____ **Where** is it?	Right here (_points to right lumbar area_).
_____ Does it **radiate**?	A little into my right leg.

Intensity

_____ On a **scale** from 1 to 10, with 10 being the worst pain, how would it rate?	A 5.

Exacerbation

_____ What makes it **worse**?	When I bend over or twist.

Remission

_____ What makes it **better**?	Not moving. Ibuprofen made it a little better.
_____ How much did you take?	A couple of tablets?
_____ How often?	Twice, about 6 hours apart.

Symptoms associated

_____ Any **numbness, tingling**?	No.
_____ **Weakness**? _(chronic)_	No.
_____ Any **urinary or fecal incontinence**?	No.

MMASSH

_____ Do you have any other **medical conditions**?	No.
_____ What **MEDICATIONS** are you on?	Just the ibuprofen.
_____ Do have any **ALLERGIES**?	Bee stings.
_____ What reaction do you have?	It gets really swollen at the site.
_____ Have you had any **SURGERIES**?	I had my tonsils taken out.
_____ Any **hospitalizations**?	Just for my tonsils.
_____ When was the **FDLNMP**?	One week ago.

Case Review #4: 26 y/o female c/o back pain

In this case, it is very important to define the time frame including onset of pain, past incidences of the same complaint, and how the pain has changed since it first started. Abdominal pain that starts at the umbilicus and moves into the right lower quadrant is characteristic of appendicitis; hence, developing the pattern of pain is key. It is also important to identify other areas of pain and if the pain radiates anywhere. **BQ**: Pain from gallstones classically radiates into the right shoulder blade. In this case, the patient's back pain radiates into the leg, which is a sign of radiculopathy or irritation of the nerve.

Knowing what a patient is doing when pain occurs also alters the differential diagnosis. Here the patient bends over and rotates simultaneously, a position that weakens the supporting ligaments of the spinal column and risks intervertebral disc bulge or herniation.

When determining intensity, a scale must be provided for the patient. One classic pain scale is denoted as from being from 0 to 10, with 10 being the worst possible pain.

The symptoms associated reflect upon the severity and urgency of the presentation.

CASE 5
32 y/o male complaining of a sore throat

Chief Complaint (**CC**): _____

C - Chronology: _____

O - Onset:_____

D - Description: _____

　　　Duration: _____

I - Intensity: _____

E - Exacerbating Factors: _____

R - Remitting Factors: _____

S - Symptoms Associated: _____

M - Medications: _____

M - Medical History: _____

A - Allergies: _____

S - Surgical: _____

S - Social Hx: _____

H - Hospitalization Hx: _____

List three things in the Differential Diagnosis

_____

_____

_____

CASE 5
Write-Up

Date: _____

Time: _____

Chief Complaint: _____

_____

Subjective: _____

_____

_____

_____

_____

_____

Assessment: _____

_____

_____

_____

_____

_____

Plan: _____

_____

_____

_____

_____

_____

Legible Signature: _____

CASE 5
32 y/o male complaining of a sore throat

_____ Introduces self and explains role.
_____ What brings you in today?   I've got a sore throat.

Chronology/Onset

_____ **When** did it start?   About 2 days ago.
_____ How has it **changed**?   It's just getting worse and worse.
_____ Did you ever have this **before**?   Yes.
_____ **How often** does it happen?   It's been a long time since the last one.
_____ **How long ago** was that?   At least a couple of years.

Description

_____ **Describe** what it feels like.   My throat's just really scratchy.

Intensity

_____ Does it **hurt to swallow**?   Yes.

Exacerbation

_____ What makes it **worse**?   Swallowing anything at all.

Remission

_____ What makes it **better**?   That sore throat spray helps a little.

Symptoms associated

_____ Do you have a **runny nose/sinus pressure**?   Not really.
_____ Any **fever or chills**?   I have felt warm.
_____ Do you have any **cough**?   No.
_____ Do you feel **really tired**?   Not really.
_____ Do you have any **ear pain**?   No.
_____ Do you have any **abdominal pain**?   No.

MMASSH

_____ Do you have any **medical** conditions?   I have reflux.
_____ Are you on any **medications**?   I take ranitidine.
_____ Are your **symptoms controlled**?   Not all the time.
_____ Do you have any **allergies**?   No.
_____ Do you **smoke**?   No.
_____ Do you **drink alcohol**?   Yes.
_____ **How much** a day?   Not every day, maybe 2–3 a week.
_____ **How many** at a setting?   One or two.
_____ **Contact with others** with the same?   I think my girlfriend had it last week.

Case Review #5: 32 y/o male complaining of a sore throat

Again, this is a fairly straightforward case. The patient has a sore throat that has progressed in severity over the last 2 days. Intensity is imprecise, although you could ask the intensity of pain on a scale. Within the symptoms associated we pose the question of fever. Very often, patients will present with the complaint of fever; however, on further questioning, they really haven't taken their own temperature. The appropriate follow-up to the complaint of fever is to ask how high it was. Also, don't allow the patient to get away with telling you that "it's been a long time" since the last infection; clarify the time frame.

The other questions regarding symptoms associated revolve around the upper respiratory tract including the sinuses, ears, nose, and lungs. A significant complaint of fatigue may clue you into mononucleosis, as would left upper quadrant pain suggestive of splenomegaly.

Another clue may be found in his history of reflux. Reflux can cause a sore throat as well as coughing and wheezing. Finding out that the patient has reflux guides you into asking if it is controlled. An additional question could have been asked as to how often he has breakthrough symptoms.

Finally, discovering that the patient was in contact with someone who had similar complaints heightens your suspicion that we are likely talking about an infectious process.

CASE 6
13 y/o female presents complaining of abdominal pain; mother is present

one to treat the patient since [illegible]

Chief Complaint (**CC**): _____

C - Chronology: _____

O - Onset: _____

D - Description: _____

    Duration: _____

I - Intensity: _____

E - Exacerbating Factors: _____

R - Remitting Factors: _____

S - Symptoms Associated: _____

M - Medications: _____

M - Medical History: _____

A - Allergies: _____

S - Surgical: _____

S - Social Hx: _____

H - Hospitalization Hx: _____

List three things in the Differential Diagnosis

_____

_____

_____

CASE 6
Write-Up

Date: _____

Time: _____

Chief Complaint: _____

_____

Subjective: _____

_____

_____

_____

_____

_____

Assessment: _____

_____

_____

_____

_____

Plan: _____

_____

_____

_____

_____

Legible Signature: _____

CASE 6
13 y/o female presents complaining of abdominal pain; her mother is present

_____	Introduction.	
_____	What brings you in today?	My belly hurts.

Chronology

_____	Have you had this before?	No.
_____	Have there been any changes in the pain?	Yes. It started at my belly button and now it's down here (points RLQ).

Onset

_____	**When** did it **start**?	Yesterday afternoon.
_____	What were you **doing**?	Watching TV.

Description/Duration

_____	**Describe** the pain.	It's real sharp and burning.
_____	**Where** is it?	Points to RLQ.
_____	Does it **radiate (go)** anywhere?	No.
_____	Is it constant or does it come and go?	Constant.

Intensity

_____	How severe is it, on a scale from **1 to 10**?	An 11.

Exacerbation

_____	What makes it **worse**?	Touching my belly or moving.

Remission

_____	Did you try anything to make it **better**?	Tylenol, but it didn't help.
_____	How much did you take?	Mom just gave me a couple tablets.

Symptoms associated

_____	Any **burning** with urination?	No.
_____	Any **fever or chills**?	I didn't take it, but I feel warm.
_____	Any **nausea or vomiting**?	I'm a little nauseated.
_____	Any **vaginal discharge or bleeding**?	No.
_____	Do you have any **diarrhea**?	A little.
_____	Was there any **blood or mucous**?	No.
_____	Felt hungry/anorexia?	No, I don't feel like eating.

MMASSH

_____	Do you have any other **medical conditions**?	No.
_____	Are you on any **MEDICATIONS**?	No.
_____	Do have any **ALLERGIES**?	No.
_____	Have you had any **SURGERIES**?	No.
_____	Any **hospitalizations**?	No.

Sexual Hx

_____	Are you **sexually active**?	I don't think so.
_____	When was the **FDLNMP**?	I don't know.
_____	Have you had your first **period** yet?	Yes.
_____	When was that?	When I was 12.
_____	Did you have a period in the last month?	I think so.

Case Review #6: 13 y/o female presents complaining of abdominal pain; mother is present

In this Flow, we again have an adolescent patient. However, in this case, she is quite adept at answering her own questions. You'll be surprised how many times a parent will try to tell you what their child's pain feels like. The patient was watching television when the pain started, which lessens the concern for trauma. The most important question in this Flow is found in how the pain has changed. **BQ:** The classic presentation for appendicitis is onset of pain around the umbilicus with progression to the right lower quadrant (RLQ). (See Appendix B for abbreviations.)

As we offer pain scales and explain the meaning, you will still find patients who respond with a number that is outside of the scale. In this case, if you could see the patient's fetal position and facial expression, you would doubt very little that she really means 11 out of 10. I have had other patients who say it's a 15 with a smile on their face. A good tool for clarification in these cases where you doubt sincerity is to define 10 out of 10 as pain that is so bad it would require hospitalization.

The abdominal pain is worse with movement or touching it, which suggests possible peritoneal signs.

The symptoms associated include some of the other classic signs of appendicitis. Thinking of other organ systems in the right lower quadrant, we include the colon by asking about diarrhea. With an affirmative answer, we question further to ask about blood or mucous: Could she have inflammatory bowel disease or infectious colitis?

We should also consider female reproductive organs. Here we run into a small road block. With mom in the room, it may be hard to re-address her indecision as to whether she is sexually active. It may just be her level of understanding, thinking perhaps that kissing boys is sexual activity. In the Flow, you are allowed to get away with not pursuing the answer; however, this is a good example of where our prior discussion of interviewing adolescents alone may come in handy. Here, I would ask the patient if she understands what I mean by being sexually active. If I believed that she did not understand, I would ask if she knew what sex was. Most 13-year-olds will indeed know. There is a fine line to be walked. Asking mom if she has had any discussions with her daughter may help you to grasp the patient's level of understanding.

Another stumbling block is reached when asking her FDLNMP. Maybe she just truly doesn't keep tract of it. First ask if she has had her first period. If she hasn't, maybe she has an imperforate hymen and is having her first menses now, which would result in the pain she is having. If she has been menstruating, try to narrow down the time frame to rule out pregnancy. No matter what she tells you, you'll be doing a pregnancy test in any case.

CASE 7
24 y/o male c/o mole

Chief Complaint (**CC**): _____

C - Chronology: _____

O - Onset:_____

D - Description: _____

    Duration: _____

I - Intensity: _____

E - Exacerbating Factors: _____

R - Remitting Factors: _____

S - Symptoms Associated: _____

M - Medications: _____

M - Medical History: _____

A - Allergies: _____

S - Surgical: _____

S - Social Hx: _____

H - Hospitalization Hx: _____

List three things in the Differential Diagnosis

_____

_____

_____

CASE 7
Write-Up

Date: _____

Time: _____

Chief Complaint: _____

_____

Subjective: _____

_____

_____

_____

_____

Assessment: _____

_____

_____

_____

_____

Plan: _____

_____

_____

_____

_____

Legible Signature: _____

CASE 7
24 y/o male c/o mole

_____ Introduction.	
_____ What brings you in today?	I have this mole my girlfriend doesn't like the color of.

Chronology/Onset

_____ **When** did you first notice it?	It's been there ever since I can remember.
_____ Has it **changed** in appearance?	She said it's bigger and has changed colors.
_____ What **color** is it?	Brown and black.

Description/Duration

_____ **Where** is it?	On my back.

Exacerbation

_____ Does anything **irritate it**?	Not really.

Symptoms associated

_____ Does it **itch**?	Maybe, a little.
_____ Does it **bleed**?	No.
_____ Have you had any **sunburns**?	Yes, a couple.
_____ Did you **blister**?	Yes, a couple of times.

Family History

_____ Any **family history of skin cancer**?	My Dad had something taken off of him.
_____ Did he require further treatment?	No.

MMASSH

_____ Any **previous medical conditions**?	No.
_____ Are you on any **MEDICATIONS**?	No.
_____ Do have any **ALLERGIES**?	No.
_____ Have you had any **SURGERIES**?	I had another mole taken off.
_____ **When**?	A couple of years ago.
_____ What did it show?	They said it was plastic.
_____ Confirm "dysplastic."	Yes, that's it.
_____ Do you **smoke**?	No.

Case Review #7: 24 y/o male c/o mole

This Flow has a very limited complaint. Notice that I have combined Chronology and Onset sections in this history. Onset is actually a subcategory of chronology. Skin lesions will have specific characteristics but vary in the way of intensity or remitting factors. If this had been a lesion other than a mole that people typically do not apply medications to, such as a rash, a remitting factor question could involve which medications were used on it and the effects of these medications. Skin lesions can change appearance with the use of topicals and yet not go away, so that when the patient presents to you or the dermatologist, knowing what the lesion looked like before treatment began can aid in accurate diagnoses.

Asking about sunburns refers to the patient's skin type. People who burn and do not tan have a higher risk of melanoma. Melanoma also has familial tendencies so that a family history of melanoma would heighten suspicion. In addition, this patient had a previous mole that looked suspicious enough to another provider to do a biopsy, which showed dysplastic changes. Again, this increases his risk of a future melanoma.

Smoking is an additive risk factor for skin cancer.

CASE 8
24 y/o female presents to the family practice office complaining of knee pain

Chief Complaint (**CC**): _____

C - Chronology: _____

O - Onset: _____

D - Description: _____

    Duration: _____

I - Intensity: _____

E - Exacerbating Factors: _____

R - Remitting Factors: _____

S - Symptoms Associated: _____

M - Medications: _____

M - Medical History: _____

A - Allergies: _____

S - Surgical: _____

S - Social Hx: _____

H - Hospitalization Hx: _____

List three things in the Differential Diagnosis

_____

_____

_____

CASE 8
Write-Up

Date: _____

Time: _____

Chief Complaint: _____

_____

Subjective: _____

_____

_____

_____

_____

_____

Assessment: _____

_____

_____

_____

_____

Plan: _____

_____

_____

_____

_____

Legible Signature: _____

CASE 8
24 y/o female presents to the family practice office complaining of knee pain

____	Introduction.	
____	What brings you in today?	I have pain in my knee.

Chronology

____	Have you **had this before**?	No.
____	Has there been any **change in the pain**?	It's been getting worse.

Onset

____	**When** did it **start**?	A week ago.
____	What were you **doing** when it started?	I just noticed it when I woke up.
____	Was there any history of **trauma**?	No.

Description/Duration

____	**Describe** the pain.	It's like an ache.
____	**Where** is it?	Points to right knee inferior patella.
____	Does it **radiate (go)** anywhere?	Not really.
____	Is it **constant** or **does it come and go**?	It's constant.

Intensity

____	How severe is it on a scale from **1 to 10**?	About a 7 or 8.

Exacerbation

____	What makes it **worse**?	If I put any weight on my leg at all.

Remission

____	Did you try anything to make it **better**?	A heating pad helped a little.

Symptoms associated

____	Any **redness**?	No.
____	Any **swelling**?	I think so.
____	Any **fever or chills**?	I have felt a little warm.
____	Any **pain with movement of the leg**?	Yes.
____	Any **sore throat or vaginal discharge**?	No.
____	Any **pain in the calf**?	No.
____	Any **SOB or chest pain**?	No.

MMASSH

____	Any other **medical conditions** you've had?	No.
____	Are you on any **MEDICATIONS**?	Birth control pill.
____	Do have any **ALLERGIES**?	No.
____	Do you **smoke**?	Yes.
____	**How much** a day?	One pack a day.
____	**How long** have you smoked?	I started when I was 16.
____	Do you **drink alcohol**?	No.
____	Have you had any **SURGERIES**?	No.
____	Any **hospitalizations**?	No.
____	When was the **FDLNMP**?	One week ago.

Case Review #8: 24 y/o female presents to the family practice office complaining of knee pain

The patient presents with isolated right knee pain and no prior history of a similar complaint or injury. Patients who present with an injury complaint, such as the football player who has a knee injury with known mechanism, limit the diagnostic possibilities to the anatomic injury that has occurred. In this case, the patient awakens with the knee pain so that we can include injury, such as if she had played tennis for the first time in 5 years the day before, but we cannot limit ourselves to it.

The pain is described as an ache of significant intensity aggravated by weight bearing. At this point the differential diagnosis would include musculoskeletal knee pain.

The bothersome part of the history is the precise fact that she has had no injury. Anatomically, what else could be causing the pain? Her young age and short duration of complaint make degenerative joint disease unlikely. Could she have rheumatoid arthritis? **BQ**: One other possibility is an infectious knee; hence, the questions of sore throat, vaginal discharge, and fever to rule out arthritis secondary to gonorrhea.

The area of pain must be questioned precisely. As we are only in the history taking stage, we limit ourselves to questions, wherein an actual clinical setting, we would simply lay our hands on the patient and discern where we elicit pain. Here, we ask specifically about calf pain, shortness of breath (SOB), and chest pain for the possibility of a deep vein thrombosis in this patient who is on birth control and smokes.

thirsty all the time
fatigue
lost 10 lbs   dark urine
2 month

CASE 9
24 y/o female c/o a urinary tract infection (UTI)

Chief Complaint (CC): ___UTI___

C - Chronology: ___yes, (last) ABT a year infection (2-15 uss) co___

O - Onset: ___2 weeks___

D - Description: ___fee all the time___

Duration: ___

I - Intensity: ___

E - Exacerbating Factors: ___no___

R - Remitting Factors: ___cranberry juice didn't work___

S - Symptoms Associated: ___no burning sensation, no pain, no bladder cramp___
no incontinence

M - Medications: ___no med___

M - Medical History: ___no other medical issues (other than UTI)___

A - Allergies: ___NKA___

S - Surgical: ___no surgery___

S - Social Hx: ___STD TX 05___ no alcohol, no drug, no tobacco, no
normal diet,

H - Hospitalization Hx: ___none___

List three things in the Differential Diagnosis ___sexually active last week + TD LMP
generally use protection

___flu___

___

___

Both parents have diabetes   allergy?

How often?   Smell/pain?

CASE 9
Write-Up

Date: _____

Time: _____

Chief Complaint: _____

_____

Subjective: _____

_____

_____

_____

_____

_____

Assessment: _____

_____

_____

_____

_____

_____

Plan: _____

_____

_____

_____

_____

Legible Signature: _____

CASE 9
24 y/o female c/o a UTI

[handwritten: urinaly culture w/?]

_____ Introduction.
_____ What brings you in today?
_____ How do you know it's a urinary tract infection?

I have a urinary tract infection.
I have to pee all the time.

[handwritten: polyurea]

[handwritten: tested for diabetes?]

[handwritten: polyurea polydypsea polyphagia]

Chronology

_____ Have you had urinary tract infections before?
_____ When was the last one?
_____ What did they do for you then?

Yes.
A couple of years ago.
They gave me an antibiotic and a yeast infection.

Onset

_____ **When** did you first notice it?

It's been a couple of weeks now.

Description/Duration

_____ **What symptoms** are you having?
_____ **How often** is "all the time?"

I just pee all the time.
It seems like every half an hour.

Exacerbation

_____ Does anything make it worse?

Not really.

Remission

_____ Did you try anything to make it better?

Cranberry juice, but it didn't work.

Symptoms associated

_____ Do you have any **burning** with urination?
_____ Do you have any **blood** with urination?
_____ Are you **thirsty** or **hungry** a lot?
_____ Any **lightheadedness or dizziness**?
_____ Any **weight loss or gain**?
_____ Over what **period of time**?
_____ Any **fatigue**?

No.
No.
Yes, I am thirsty all the time.
No.
I've actually lost about 10 lbs.
Two months.
I seem to be tired all the time.

[handwritten: polydypsea polydypsea]

[handwritten: at night? 10 yo meadose, 10 no → DRINKS too much]

MMASSH

_____ Any **previous medical conditions**?
_____ Are you on any **MEDICATIONS**?
_____ Do have any **ALLERGIES**?
_____ Have you had any **SURGERIES**?
_____ Any **hospitalizations**?

No.
No.
No.
No.
No.

[handwritten: unprescribed diuretics?]

Social History

_____ Are you **sexually active**?
_____ Do you use **protection**?
_____ When was the **FDLNMP**?

Yes.
Yes.
Last week.

Family History

_____ Does anyone in your family have diabetes?

Both my mother and my father.

Case Review #9: 24 y/o female c/o a UTI

Be wary of the patient who presents with a diagnosis in hand for you. In some cases, it may be helpful, like the young man presenting in the emergency room with abdominal pain and known inflammatory bowel disease. He had been through this type of pain many times and knew exactly what was happening again. Those who study medicine also present with proposed diagnoses. It is rather coincidental that many don't discover their maladies until they move to that section in their studies. The proposed diagnosis may be included in your differential as the patient is often correct, but it should not limit the other possibilities. The remainder of your questions should prove or disprove the patient.

When this patient stated she had a "urinary tract infection," the immediate next question was, "How do you know it's a urinary tract infection?" This allowed the patient to state symptoms she had that she believed were caused by a UTI. She could have as easily said she knew because she has had them in the past, which would have directed you to ask her for the specific symptoms of a urinary tract infection she had earlier.

Her isolated complaint of urinary frequency was the clue that something else may be going on. Urinary tract infections rarely present with just urinary frequency, having instead the associated dysuria, hematuria, and suprapubic discomfort.

So, at this point you have to ask yourself what else causes someone to urinate all the time. I must admit that I had inside information on this patient, as I already was treating both of her parents for diabetes. In addition, I had the added benefit of being able to see her body habitus, which increased her risk for diabetes.

Suspecting diabetes, you then ask about symptoms associated such as polydipsia, polyphagia, fatigue, and weight loss.

The sexual/social history correlates with urinary tract infections, which are more common in people who are sexually active.

Finally, take the hint from the patient about the outcome of her last treatment with antibiotics. She obviously wasn't happy with the resultant yeast infection. Are patients with diabetes more prone to yeast infections? Add another clue.

CASE 10
26 y/o female c/o a cold

Chief Complaint (CC): _____

C - Chronology: _____

O - Onset: _____

D - Description: _____

    Duration: _____

I - Intensity: _____

E - Exacerbating Factors: _____

R - Remitting Factors: _____

S - Symptoms Associated: _____

M - Medications: _____

M - Medical History: _____

A - Allergies: _____

S - Surgical: _____

S - Social Hx: _____

H - Hospitalization Hx: _____

List three things in the Differential Diagnosis

_____

_____

_____

CASE 10
Write-Up

Date: _____

Time: _____

Chief Complaint: _____

_____

Subjective: _____

_____

_____

_____

_____

_____

Assessment: _____

_____

_____

_____

_____

Plan: _____

_____

_____

_____

_____

Legible Signature: _____

CASE 10
26 y/o female c/o a cold

Chronology

_____ Introduction.

_____ What brings you in today? — I've got a cold.

_____ Did you ever have this **before**? — Yes.

_____ **How often** does it happen? — About once a year.

Onset

_____ **When** did it start? — About 3 days ago.

Description/Duration

_____ What **symptoms** are you having? — A runny nose, sore throat and cough.

_____ Did they all start at the same time? — No. I had a runny nose first, then the sore throat and cough today.

_____ What **color** is the drainage from your nose? — It was clear, but now it's green.

_____ **Bringing anything up** with the cough? — Yes, a little.

_____ What **color** is it? — I don't know. I don't look at it.

Intensity

_____ Have you **missed work/school**? — Yes, I took off yesterday.

Exacerbation

_____ What makes it **worse**? — Coughing makes my throat worse.

Remission

_____ What makes it **better**? — A shower clears my nose a little.

_____ Did you try any **medications** for your cold? — I took some TheraFlu.

_____ Did it help? — Just a little.

Symptoms associated

_____ Do you have any **sinus congestion/pressure**? — Yes.

_____ Any **fever or chills**? — No.

_____ Do you have any **SOB**? — No.

_____ **Vomiting or diarrhea**? — No.

_____ **Eating and drinking** all right? — Yes.

_____ Any **ear pain**? — No.

MMASSH

_____ Do you have any **medical** conditions? — No.

_____ Are you on any **medications**? — No.

_____ Do you have any **allergies**? — No.

_____ Do you **smoke**? — Yes.

_____ **How much a day**? — A pack a day for 10 years.

_____ Do you normally have a **cough**? — No.

_____ When was the **FDLNMP**? — It started yesterday.

_____ **Contact** to others with similar symptoms? — Yes, my sister had the same thing last week.

Case Review #10: 26 y/o female c/o a cold

When this patient presents with a "cold," the real job is to define whether a cold to this patient means otitis, sinusitis, pharyngitis, or bronchitis, and then basing your treatment decision on a viral or bacterial etiology.

Time frame is important. Here, we note that the first symptom was rhinorrhea that has indeed changed from a clear discharge to one which is green, suggesting a bacterial component. The rhinorrhea is associated with sinus pressure and we could quantify the amount of exudate. Frequently, patients will describe clear rhinorrhea that later becomes thickened and green, resulting in nasal congestion and sinus pressure with possible sinusitis. Pediatric patients may develop exudate from the eyes, which may be ascension through the nasolacrimal duct.

The sore throat is likely from post-nasal drainage as the runny nose started first and then the sore throat, but pharyngitis remains in the differential diagnosis. No other organ systems seem to be involved to any great extent.

Notice that we try to get a description of the expectorant. Be aware that some patients will be less than willing to give a description, while others may take great pleasure in describing the color, consistency, etc. in great detail.

The patient had contact with someone with similar symptoms, although that person often gets better as this patient suffers. It's also a great time to advise her to quit smoking as these infections are much more common in smokers.

Make appt for her w/ ob gyn

High Risk Pregnancy

CASE 11
18 y/o pregnant female presents to the ER with burning on urination

Chief Complaint (CC): bladder infection

C - Chronology: 2x before (when 15 years)

O - Onset: 2 weeks (sudden urge to urinate, burning upon urination)

D - Description: burning when it starts

Duration: constant (not just when she pees)

I - Intensity:

E - Exacerbating Factors: when peeing   FOL UP → DS Mos ago

R - Remitting Factors: N/A

S - Symptoms Associated: no back pain, no pain in abdomen, no fever/chills, no bloating, no vomiting/diarrhea

M - Medications: no

M - Medical History: 9 mos pregnant, 1st child, never approved, no reg checkups, no prenatal vitamins

A - Allergies: No allergies

S - Surgical: no surgery

S - Social Hx: used to be a carrier, not married, feels safe, trusts him, been together 2 years, [illegible], school to be [illegible], see family every [illegible]

H - Hospitalization Hx: none

normal diet, trying staying active, no caffeine, no tobacco products, no drugs, been sexually active since pregnancy, no protection, only partner

List three things in the Differential Diagnosis

UTI

STD

Herpes

been sexually active

have sex more often (2x a day)

urine is a little red

clear drainage → 2 weeks ago, no odor
no lesions/dryness   had STD before — chlamydia
no blood in urine.   15 years (treated it) resolve symptoms

CASE 11
Write-Up

Date: _____

Time: _____

Chief Complaint: _____

_____

Subjective: _____

_____

_____

_____

_____

Assessment: _____

_____

_____

_____

_____

Plan: _____

_____

_____

_____

_____

Legible Signature: _____

CASE 11
18 y/o pregnant female presents to the ER with burning on urination

_____ Introduction.	
_____ What brings you in today?	I have a bladder infection.

Chronology/Onset

_____ **When** did it **start**?	About 2 weeks ago.
_____ Have you had urinary tract infections **before**?	Yes, twice.
_____ **When** were they?	When I was 15.

Description/Duration

_____ What **symptoms** are you having now?	I have a lot burning down there.

Exacerbation

_____ What makes it **worse**?	When I pee.

Remission

_____ Did you try anything to make it **better**?	No.

Symptoms associated

_____ Are you urinating more **frequently**?	No.
_____ Any problems **getting it started**?	Yea, because it burns when it starts.
_____ Do you have any **urgency**?	Yea, I'd like to get out of here.
_____ Do you get sudden **urges** to urinate?	No.
_____ Any **fever or chills**?	No.
_____ Any **abdominal or back pain**?	No.
_____ Any **nausea or vomiting**?	No.
_____ Do you have any **vaginal discharge or bleeding**?	Just a little clear drainage.
_____ Do you have any **lesions** in the genital area?	I didn't look.

OB/GYN history

_____ How many **weeks pregnant** are you?	About 4 months.
_____ When was the **FDLNMP**?	About 5 months ago.
_____ How many **times** have you been **pregnant**?	This is the first time.
_____ Do you have an OB/GYN doctor?	No, I just moved here.

Sexual Hx

_____ Are you **sexually active**?	I'm pregnant, aren't I?
_____ Are you sexually active during your pregnancy?	Yes.
_____ Does your **partner** have any **discharge or lesions**?	He's a little raw. He says he's not used to having sex so often.
_____ Is he your only partner?	Yes.
_____ Do you use **protection**?	No, I'm pregnant. And I trust him.

(continues)

	How long have you been with him?	About a month.
	Have you ever had a **sexually transmitted disease**?	I had chlamydia once.
	When was that?	When I was 15.

MMASSH

	Are you on any **MEDICATIONS**?	No.
	Are you taking prenatal vitamins?	No.
	Do have any **ALLERGIES**?	No.
	Have you had any **SURGERIES**?	No.
	Any **hospitalizations**?	No.
	Any other **medical conditions** you've had?	No.

Case Review #11: 18 y/o pregnant female presents to the ER with burning on urination

This case is nearly word for word for what really happened in my practice. There were more questions to this case than I could include, but essentially the young lady had come from another town and recently moved into the area. Her chief complaint was burning with urination, and she also had the ready diagnosis of an UTI, exactly like our other patient.

This case was a little trickier than the last because she truly did have dysuria; however, the key to the case was that she said she had burning all of the time, not just when she urinated, which was not consistent with typical UTIs. She also lacked frequency, urgency, fever, chills, abdominal or back pain.

This case demonstrates the importance of speaking on the correct level with the patient. She obviously did not know what "urgency" meant. In fact, her exact words were "Yea, I waited 2 hours and I want to get the _____ out of here". The important thing is not to walk away from the question, but to rephrase it so that it is understood.

An extensive OB/GYN history is important as the patient has not had prenatal care. Estimate the gestational age by asking for the FDLNMP. This is where the "N" from the abbreviation becomes important in that gestational age may be miscalculated if based on a menses that was not normal for the patient.

The burning without urination makes one concerned about a sexually transmitted disease (STD), specifically herpes simplex. The patient has not looked for lesions; however, one can still ask about burning or tingling in the area, which are symptoms typical before the onset of lesions secondary to herpes simplex virus.

A detailed sexual history shows the patient has a new partner and continues to have unprotected sex. Unfortunately, the exam confirmed the suspicion and she was informed that the partner she "trusts" just gave her herpes. She might have to have a caesarean section if she had a current outbreak when she was in labor. His being "raw" was most likely an active herpes outbreak. Although such frank language is not perhaps typical, the provider must develop a sense of composure. Some patients intentionally go for the shock effect as part of their persona.

This patient was referred to an OB/GYN with an appointment that afternoon; unfortunately, she failed to show for the appointment.

CASE 12
24 y/o male medical student presents to the family practice office c/o chest pain

Chief Complaint (**CC**): _____

C - Chronology: _____

O - Onset: _____

D - Description: _____

　　　Duration: _____

I - Intensity: _____

E - Exacerbating Factors: _____

R - Remitting Factors: _____

S - Symptoms Associated: _____

M - Medications: _____

M - Medical History: _____

A - Allergies: _____

S - Surgical: _____

S - Social Hx: _____

H - Hospitalization Hx: _____

List three things in the Differential Diagnosis

_____

_____

_____

CASE 12
Write-Up

Date: _____

Time: _____

Chief Complaint: _____

_____

Subjective: _____

_____

_____

_____

_____

_____

Assessment: _____

_____

_____

_____

_____

Plan: _____

_____

_____

_____

_____

Legible Signature: _____

CASE 12
24 y/o male medical student presents to the family practice office complaining of chest pain

_____ Introduction.
_____ What brings you in today? I have chest pain.

Chronology/Onset

_____ **When** did it **start**? A couple of months ago.
_____ What are you **doing** when it occurs? It's usually after I eat.
_____ Have there been any **changes in the pain**? It's been getting more frequent.
_____ Have you had this **before**? No.

Description/Duration

_____ **Describe** the pain. It's like a burning.
_____ **Where** is it? Points to epigastria.
_____ Does it **radiate (go)** anywhere? Sometimes a little up into my neck.
_____ Is it **constant** or **come and go**? It comes and goes.
_____ How long does it **last**? A couple of hours.

Intensity

_____ How severe is it on a scale from **1 to 10**? About a 4 or 5.

Exacerbation

_____ What makes it **worse**? If I eat before going to bed or have certain foods.
_____ What **kinds of foods**? Spicy stuff.

Remission

_____ Did you try anything to make it **better**? Mylanta helps for about an hour.

Symptoms associated

_____ Any **sweating**? No.
_____ Any **abdominal or back pain**? No.
_____ Any **nausea or vomiting**? I'm a little nauseated sometimes.
_____ Any **diarrhea or constipation**? No.
_____ Any **blood or dark colored stools**? No.

MMASSH

_____ Any other **medical conditions** you've had? Asthma, when I was a kid.
_____ Are you on any **MEDICATIONS**? No.
_____ Do have any **ALLERGIES**? No.
_____ Do you **smoke**? No.
_____ Do you **drink alcohol**? Yes.
_____ **How much** a week? I have about 3 beers a week.
_____ Do you use any **drugs**? No way.
_____ Have you had any **SURGERIES**? No.
_____ Any **hospitalizations**? No.

Case Review #12: 24 y/o male medical student presents to the family practice office complaining of chest pain

Notice how the complaint of chest pain brings to mind a markedly different differential diagnosis in a 24-year-old than in a 64-year-old. Before asking your first question, you should have already moved myocardial infarction way down on your list. Is it still possible? Of course it is, but it is much less likely.

This flow demonstrates the power of an accurate chronological history. If you didn't follow-up the onset by asking what he was doing when it occurred, you would have missed that it occurs after eating. Top on our list of possibilities becomes cholelithiasis, gastroesophageal reflux, and peptic or duodenal ulcer disease. His description of the pain as "burning" conforms. Do not be fooled by this characteristic. Cardiac pain can be described as burning in nature.

True Story

A middle aged colleague was walking up a flight of stairs. When he reached the top, he complained about having heartburn. It was a short encounter but, in retrospect, walking up stairs is not a common aggravating factor for dyspepsia. One week later the gentleman had cardiac bypass.

BQ: Regarding location, the pain pattern of radiation is particularly helpful as cholelithiasis classically radiates in the right shoulder blade, a dissecting aneurysm into the back, and reflux often centrally into the neck and throat.

When asking about exacerbating factors, follow through for more details. When you find out that food makes the symptoms worse, ask what kind of food. If dairy products were involved, we would have to add lactose intolerance to our differential and ask about the appropriate symptoms associated with it. What happens when we go to bed shortly after eating? The supine position encourages reflux.

Finally, determining alcohol intake gives you the opportunity to educate your patient. Inform them that alcohol and tobacco loosen the gastroesophageal sphincter. So if you have glass of wine before you go to bed, not only are you in the proper position to more gastric acid flow up into the esophagus, but you also relax the sphincter to allow gastric fluid through.

CASE 13
32 y/o male presents with SOB

Chief Complaint (**CC**): _____

C - Chronology: _____

O - Onset:_____

D - Description: _____

     Duration: _____

I - Intensity: _____

E - Exacerbating Factors: _____

R - Remitting Factors: _____

S - Symptoms Associated: _____

M - Medications: _____

M - Medical History: _____

A - Allergies: _____

S - Surgical: _____

S - Social Hx: _____

H - Hospitalization Hx: _____

List three things in the Differential Diagnosis

_____

_____

_____

CASE 13
Write-Up

Date: _____

Time: _____

Chief Complaint: _____

_____

Subjective: _____

_____

_____

_____

_____

_____

Assessment: _____

_____

_____

_____

_____

Plan: _____

_____

_____

_____

_____

Legible Signature: _____

CASE 13
32 y/o male presents with SOB

_____ Introduction.
_____ What brings you in today?   I can't catch my breath.

Chronology/Onset
_____ **When** did it start?   Last night.
_____ **What are you doing** when it occurs?   I was playing basketball.
_____ Did it start **suddenly or gradually**?   I was a little short of breath when I was
                                                      playing, but then it got suddenly worse.
_____ Has it **changed** since last night?   It's getting harder and harder to breathe.
_____ Did you ever have this **before**?   No.

Description/Duration
_____ Is it **constant** or does it **come and go**?   It's constant.

Intensity
_____ Do you feel **lightheaded**?   No.
_____ Has it affected your **sleep**?   I woke up a lot last night short of breath.
_____ Were you able to finish the game?   No, I quit early.

Exacerbation
_____ What makes it **worse**?   It's worse when I exert myself or if I lay on my
                                                      right side.

Remission
_____ What makes it **better**?   Nothing.

Symptoms associated
_____ Have you had **a cold** recently?   No.
_____ Any **wheezing**?   No.
_____ Do you have any chest **pain**?   Only when I felt a pop when it first started.
       _____ **Where** is the pain?   Here in my left chest (points to left upper thorax).
       _____ **How long** did it last?   Only a few seconds.
_____ Do you have a **cough**?   Yes.
_____ Are you bringing up any **sputum**?   A little.
       _____ What **color** is it?   Clear.
_____ Did you bring up any blood?   Maybe a little streak of it.

MMASSH
_____ Do you have any **medical conditions**?   No.
_____ History of **lung disease/asthma**?   I had asthma as a kid.
_____ Are you on any **MEDICATIONS**?   No.
_____ Do have any **ALLERGIES**?   No.
_____ Have you had any **SURGERIES**?   No.
_____ Do you **smoke**?   When I'm out with the guys.
       _____ How much in a week?   Probably 6 cigarettes a month.
_____ Any **hospitalizations**?   No.

Case Review #13: 32 y/o male presents with SOB

By this Case, the questions should be coming to you more naturally. When this patient presents with shortness of breath (SOB), you naturally want to know when it started and how it has changed since starting. Again, what the patient was doing is important. Playing basketball is typically a strenuous activity requiring a high cardiopulmonary output. Hence, we think of these organ systems first in our differential.

Considering the respiratory system, it is unlikely that the patient is suffering from pneumonia or any infectious process as the onset was so sudden. He could have a pulmonary embolism but he lacks leg pain, swelling, or redness associated with a deep vein thrombosis that is the most common cause of pulmonary embolism. Interestingly, the patient felt a pop in his chest associated with some pain: spontaneous pneumothorax.

Shortness of breath is difficult to assign an intensity level. It should be reflected in what activity is and is not able to be done. Here the patient could not sleep well and, more importantly, could not finish the basketball game.

Concerning the possibility of spontaneous pneumothorax, the patient heard and felt the pop in his left chest. Why would his breathing be worse when he was lying on his right side? The reason is that the patient is dependent on the right lung for his respirations, so lying on the right side essentially restricts the ability to expand the right hemithorax.

Notice the follow-up questions to the inquiry of chest pain. The patient tells you when it occurred, so you have to ask him where it occurred and its duration. You basically perform another mini CODIERS on the pain itself.

CASE 14
58 y/o female c/o swelling in her leg

Chief Complaint (**CC**): _____

C - Chronology: _____

O - Onset:_____

D - Description: _____

    Duration: _____

I - Intensity: _____

E - Exacerbating Factors: _____

R - Remitting Factors: _____

S - Symptoms Associated: _____

M - Medications: _____

M - Medical History: _____

A - Allergies: _____

S - Surgical: _____

S - Social Hx: _____

H - Hospitalization Hx: _____

List three things in the Differential Diagnosis

_____

_____

_____

CASE 14
Write-Up

Date: _____

Time: _____

Chief Complaint: _____

_____

Subjective: _____

_____

_____

_____

_____

_____

Assessment: _____

_____

_____

_____

_____

_____

Plan: _____

_____

_____

_____

_____

_____

Legible Signature: _____

CASE 14
58 y/o female c/o swelling in her leg

_____ Introduction.	
_____ What brings you in today?	I have swelling in my leg.

Chronology/Onset

_____ When did it **start**?	Three days ago.
_____ What were you **doing at the time**?	Putting my shoes on.
_____ Did you ever **have this before**?	No.
_____ How has it **changed**?	It has gotten bigger.

Description/Duration

_____ **Where** is the swelling?	It's my right leg, from my thigh down.

Intensity

_____ How bad is the swelling?	I can't get my shoe on, I'm wearing my slipper.

Exacerbation

_____ What makes it **worse**?	It gets worse as the day goes on.

Remission

_____ Does anything make it **better**?	No.

Symptoms associated

_____ Any **pain**?	Yes.
_____ **Describe** the pain.	It's a dull ache.
_____ Is it the all the time (**constant**)?	Yes.
_____ Is your leg **red**?	Yes, a little.
_____ Any **trauma**?	I did scratch it last week in the garden.
_____ Any **shortness of breath**?	No.
_____ Any **chest pain**?	No.

MMASSH

_____ Do you have any other **medical conditions**?	I get migraines now and then.
_____ What **MEDICATIONS** are you on?	None. I just take estrogen.
_____ Do have any **ALLERGIES**?	No.
_____ Do you **smoke**?	Not any more.
_____ When did you **quit**?	I quit 2 weeks ago.
_____ **How much** did you smoke before?	A pack a day.
_____ **How long** did you smoke?	Maybe 40 years.
_____ Any **recent travel**?	I visited my sister last week.
_____ How far is that away?	Oh, about a 4-hour drive.
_____ Have you had any **SURGERIES**?	I had my tonsils taken out when I was kid.
_____ Any **hospitalizations**?	No.
_____ When was the **FDLNMP**?	Oh, Honey, I don't have one of those anymore.

Case Review #14: 58 y/o female c/o swelling in her leg

This 58-year-old female presents with swelling in her leg. Without asking another question, the differential diagnosis includes cellulitis, heart failure, venous insufficiency, deep vein thrombosis (DVT), and gout, just to name a few.

The swelling has been getting progressively worse and was noticed simply because she could not get her shoe on, eliminating significant trauma as a cause. The swelling gets worse as the day goes on, supporting venous insufficiency or an obstructive process. Perhaps she has a pelvic malignancy causing lymphatic drainage compromise. She has no shortness of breath as would be likely found with congestive heart failure (CHF), and the swelling is unilateral whereas in CHF it is usually bilateral. If the patient had admitted to SOB, we would have pursued questions of orthopnea, dyspnea on exertion, and paroxysmal nocturnal dyspnea.

Your concern for cellulitis is heightened when you learn she scratched her leg in the garden a week prior. Another common entry sight is fungal infections of the toe nails.

Knowing the patient is on estrogen raises your concern for a DVT. Recent travel is additive to your suspicion. You must ask the means of travel and its duration. A 1-hour car trip is less worrisome than a 4-hour trip.

The patient's smoking history could easily have been missed. When asked if she smoked, she responded, "Not any more," leading you to ask when she had quit. If she had simply said, "No," then you may have missed it. A better question to ask is, "Have you ever smoked?" Then determine when they quit, how long they had smoked prior to quitting, and how much a day they smoked. The standard way to document smoking history is in pack-years. Pack-years are determined by multiplying the number of packs per day, by the number of years the patient smoked. For instance:

$\frac{1}{2}$ pack per day for 20 years = 10 pack-years

1 pack per day for 50 years = 50 pack-years

3 packs per day for 30 years = 90 pack-years

Along this same line, perhaps an even better question would be to ask if the patient uses tobacco at all. I have documented patient as nonsmoking only to learn later that they chew a can of snuff a day, which increases their risk for mouth and throat cancer.

You frequently will not know the exact diagnosis when you have finished gathering your history and performing your exam. You job now is to investigate each possibility to arrive at the correct diagnosis.

CASE 16
46 y/o cm presents to the ER with abdominal pain at 0200

_____ Introduction.	
_____ What brings you in today?	My stomach really hurts. ✓

Chronology/Onset

_____ When did it **start**?	Last night. ✓
_____ What were you **doing**?	Watching television. ✓
_____ Has the **pain changed** since it started?	It's just gotten worse. ✓
_____ Did you ever **have this before**?	A couple of times. ✓
_____ **When**?	About twice in the last year. It just went away on its own after a couple of days. ✓

Description/Duration

_____ What does it **feel like**?	An ache. ✓
_____ Is it constant or does it **come and go**?	It's always there, but gets worse and then better. ✓
_____ Did it come on **suddenly or gradually**?	Gradually.

Location

_____ Where is it?	In my stomach. ✓
_____ Can you show me (with one finger)?	Points to RUQ. ✓
_____ Does it radiate anywhere?	It seems to go a little into my back. ✓
_____ Where in your back?	Between my shoulder blades. ✓

Intensity

_____ On a **scale** of 1 to 10 where is it now?	An 8. ✓

Exacerbation

_____ What makes it **worse**?	I don't know. ✓
_____ Does any type of **food** make it worse?	Maybe a little. ✓

Remission

_____ Does anything make it **better**?	No. ✓

Symptoms associated

_____ **Nausea or vomiting**?	Yes, I vomited a couple of times. ✓
_____ **Diarrhea or constipation**?	A little diarrhea. ✓
_____ **Heartburn**?	No. ✓
_____ Change in **color** in the **stools**?	I don't think so. ✓
_____ **Fever, chills**?	I get hot and cold. ✓
_____ Have you noticed your **eyes being yellow**?	My wife said that they were. ✓
_____ When did she tell you that?	For about a month now. ✓
_____ Any **color change to the urine**?	It sort of looks like tea. ✓

(continues)

MMASSH

_____	Any past **Medical Conditions**?	I have high cholesterol.
_____	What **MEDICATIONS** are you on?	Only a cholesterol medication, a statin?
	_____ When did you start that?	About a month ago.
_____	Do have any **ALLERGIES**?	No
_____	Have you had any **SURGERIES**?	Just my appendix when I was a kid.
_____	Any **hospitalizations**?	Only when I was shot in the leg in Vietnam.
_____	Do you smoke?	No.
_____	Do you drink alcohol?	I have a beer now and then.
_____	Have you **traveled** anywhere?	We were in Mexico 2 months ago.
	_____ Did you get sick then?	We both got a little diarrhea for a few days.

Case Review #16:
46 y/o cm presents to the ER with abdominal pain at 0200

There is a lot of information in this case and as soon as you think you know what is going on, it changes on you; even the time that the patient came in to the ER is a clue. Most patients don't come to the ER at 2 o'clock in the morning unless they really consider their symptoms to be serious. This does not always hold true, as I distinctly remember being called to the ER early one morning to evaluate a 73-year-old man for back pain. It was the same pain that he suffered with for the last 23 years. When asked why he came in at 2 o'clock in the morning, thinking that perhaps it had gotten suddenly worse or had somehow changed, he just stated that he thought he would ask someone else about it as no one really knew what was going on for the last 23 years.

Here, there is some prior history of the same pain which the patient admits to having twice in the last year, but apparently did not seek intervention as it went away. Put gastritis, reflux, peptic ulcer disease, cholelithiasis, and even dissecting aneurysm on the differential. The pain is in the right upper quadrant and radiates to the back, not exactly to the right shoulder blade but more between the shoulder blades. Again, consider dissecting aneurysm and cholelithiasis.

The patient has vomited and you hopefully asked more detail about when the last occurrence was and what it looked like.

A method used to establish a differential diagnosis is to consider anatomy. This patient has pain in the right upper quadrant. If you pointed to the site and went straight through the body, what organ systems could be affected? First considerations are the skin and subcutaneous tissues, as herpetic zoster is a very painful condition. Look for lesions. Next the inferior anterior rib cage. Could this patient have a somatic rib dysfunction that could lead to musculoskeletal pain? Next, we hit the liver and gallbladder; consider any condition that would involve these organs such as cholelithiasis and hepatitis. The transverse bowel and descending small bowel also lie in the area: could this be colitis or duodenal ulcer? Even the inferior lobe of the right lung may be encountered with our straight line. Could pneumonia be possible?

Now, with these possibilities, ask the appropriate questions. The patient admits that his wife has noticed his eyes were yellow. We should ask here if he has ever had that before. Perhaps he has a metabolic disorder in the processing of bilirubin for elimination, like Gilbert disease. This seems unlikely in this case, so question yourself as to acute causes of hyperbilirubinemia, witnessed by icterus, yellow eyes, and tea-colored urine. Is he hemolyzing red blood cells such as that which could occur with splenomegaly? Is the bile duct obstructed by a stone or tumor? Does he have hepatitis?

The importance of MMASSH is seen here. We find out the gentleman has hyperlipidemia and that he was started on a cholesterol pill not long ago. "Aha!" We think we have our answer: drug-induced hepatotoxicity. But if we had stopped questioning and not gone a little further, we may not have found his risk for infectious hepatitis by his recent travel to Mexico.

You have your work cut out for you trying to find out which is the real diagnosis.

NOTES:

CASE 17
65 y/o female c/o dizziness

Chief Complaint (CC): _____

C - Chronology: _____

O - Onset: _____

D - Description: _____

    Duration: _____

I - Intensity: _____

E - Exacerbating Factors: _____

R - Remitting Factors: _____

S - Symptoms Associated: _____

M - Medications: _____

M - Medical History: _____

A - Allergies: _____

S - Surgical: _____

S - Social Hx: _____

H - Hospitalization Hx: _____

List three things in the Differential Diagnosis

_____

_____

_____

CASE 17
Write-Up

Date: _____

Time: _____

Chief Complaint: _____

_____

Subjective: _____

_____

_____

_____

_____

_____

Assessment: _____

_____

_____

_____

_____

_____

Plan: _____

_____

_____

_____

_____

Legible Signature: _____

CASE 17
65 y/o female c/o dizziness

_____ Introduction.	
_____ What brings you in today?	I've been dizzy.

Chronology/Onset

_____ **When** did it start?	It's been going on for about a month.
_____ **What are you doing** when it occurs?	Mostly when I stand up.
_____ Did you ever have this **before**?	No.
_____ **How often** does it happen?	At first only once a week, but now it's daily.

Description/Duration

_____ **Describe** the dizziness.	It feels like the room is closing in on me and getting darker like I'm going to pass out.
_____ Does the **room spin**?	No.
_____ **How long** does it last?	Maybe 10 or 15 minutes.

Intensity

_____ Have you **fallen or passed out**?	No.

Exacerbation

_____ What makes it **worse**?	Standing up too fast.

Remission

_____ What makes it **better**?	If I get out of bed or stand up slowly or sit back down for a few minutes.

Symptoms associated

_____ Have you had **a cold** recently?	No.
_____ Does your **heart beat fast**?	Yes, when I feel dizzy.
_____ **Vomiting or diarrhea**?	No.
_____ **Eating and drinking** well?	Yes.
_____ Any **heartburn or stomach pain**?	Yes, my stomach has been upset a bit lately.
_____ Any **blood black colored stools**?	Yes, now that you mention it, they are dark.
_____ Change in **caliber or size** of your stools?	I don't think so.
_____ Have you **lost** any **weight**?	I think I've lost a little weight.
_____ How much, over how long?	Oh, only 5 pounds in the last year or so.

MMASSH

_____ Do you have any other **medical conditions**?	I have pretty bad arthritis and high blood pressure.
_____ History of an **ulcer**?	No.
_____ What **MEDICATIONS** are you on?	Something for my blood pressure, and ibuprofen.
_____ How much ibuprofen do you take?	Usually 3 pills, three times a day, but my arthritis has really been acting up, so I've been taking more.
_____ Do have any **ALLERGIES**?	No.
_____ Have you had any **SURGERIES**?	No.
_____ Any **hospitalizations**?	Only when my children were born.

Case Review #17: 65 y/o female c/o dizziness

This woman presents with dizziness. The first thing to ask is for the patient to describe the dizziness, having them tell what they mean by it. The room spinning around is vertigo, whereas the room getting darker and feeling as if they are going to pass out is near syncope. Often you will get a description of lightheadedness or imbalance.

The patient has had this going on for a month but the frequency is increasing, suggesting a somewhat chronic process. This patient denies the sensation of the room spinning, decreasing the likelihood of labyrinthitis, inner ear dysfunction, which is often associated with recent colds; hence, the symptom associated question.

Dizziness with standing suggests decreased cerebral perfusion such as with autonomic or carotid body dysfunction or hypovolemia. She has been eating and drinking well without nausea or vomiting, which suggests that dehydration is not likely the cause. She has had some stomach upset and dark stools. Could she be anemic? We ask about weight loss and change in caliber of stools to help rule out colon cancer as a source of blood loss. Notice the follow-up to a positive weight loss screen; ask how much and over what period of time.

The patient admits tachycardia or palpitations when the dizziness occurs. Is it because the heart is trying to increase output, or could it be an arrhythmia causing the dizziness?

So we've gotten through CODIERS and have a fairly well developed differential diagnosis. MMASSH leads us to the most likely diagnosis when we find out the patient has been overdoing it with her ibuprofen for her arthritis: nonsteroidal induced gastritis with possible gastric ulceration.

CASE 18
38 y/o female c/o diarrhea

Chief Complaint (CC): _____

C - Chronology: _____

O - Onset:_____

D - Description: _____

    Duration: _____

I - Intensity: _____

E - Exacerbating Factors: _____

R - Remitting Factors: _____

S - Symptoms Associated: _____

M - Medications: _____

M - Medical History: _____

A - Allergies: _____

S - Surgical: _____

S - Social Hx: _____

H - Hospitalization Hx: _____

List three things in the Differential Diagnosis

_____

_____

_____

CASE 18
Write-Up

Date: _____

Time: _____

Chief Complaint: _____

_____

Subjective: _____

_____

_____

_____

_____

Assessment: _____

_____

_____

_____

_____

Plan: _____

_____

_____

_____

_____

Legible Signature: _____

CASE 18
38 y/o female c/o diarrhea

_____	Introduction.	
_____	What brings you in today?	I have diarrhea.

Chronology/Onset

_____	When did it **start**?	About 3 days ago.
_____	How **many times** do you go a day?	About 6 or 7 times.
_____	When was the **last time**?	About 10 minutes ago.
_____	Did you ever **have this before**?	No.

Description/Duration

_____	**Describe** what you mean by **diarrhea**.	My stools are all watery.
_____	Was there any **blood or mucous** in it?	No.

Intensity

_____	Is there any stomach (abdominal) pain?	Yes.
_____	What is the **level** of the pain (scale 1 to 10)?	Oh, about a 3 or 4.

Exacerbation

_____	What makes it **worse**?	Nothing that I know of.

Remission

_____	Does anything make it **better**?	That pink diarrhea stuff helped a little.

Symptoms associated

_____	Any **nausea or vomiting**?	No.
_____	Any **fever or chills**?	No.
_____	Any **abdominal pain**?	I'm pretty crampy.
_____	**Where** is the pain?	Just all over my belly.

MMASSH

_____	Do you have any other **medical conditions**?	I just got over a sinus infection.
_____	What **MEDICATIONS** are you on?	Just the antibiotic for my sinuses.
_____	Do have any **ALLERGIES**?	Yes.
_____	What are you allergic to and what happens?	Ibuprofen. It really messes up my stomach.
_____	Do you **smoke**?	Yes.
_____	**How much** a day?	About a half a pack.
_____	Do you **drink**?	No.
_____	Do you use any **drugs**?	No.
_____	**Contacts** with the same symptoms?	No.
_____	Recent **travel**?	No.
_____	Eat food that was **left out** or was **undercooked**?	I was at a picnic last week.
_____	Have you had any **SURGERIES**?	I had my tonsils taken out when I was a kid.
_____	Any **hospitalizations**?	No.
_____	When was the **FDLNMP**?	I don't have one. I'm on the Depo shot.

Case Review #18: 38 y/o female c/o diarrhea

The definition of diarrhea will vary from patient to patient, so that defining the condition with the patient is important. Some patients will present complaining of diarrhea and will only have one liquid stool a day. Others may not truly have any liquid stools, but only stools that are softer than what the patient considers to be normal for them. When someone presents with diarrhea, one should ask the first occurrence, the consistency of the stools, and the frequency. Equally important is when the last episode occurred. It is common for a patient to complain of diarrhea but try to "weather the storm," and present when the clinical picture is actually improving. For example, he had six liquid stools the day before, but none so far on the day that he sees you. This affects your clinical decision-making. Perhaps you will not treat this patient with aggressive antidiarrheals but rather let it run its course naturally with supportive care, like a bland diet and increased liquids only.

Acute diarrhea is often viral in nature and requires little diagnostic work-up beyond the history and physical examination. Chronic diarrhea, however, may require an extensive evaluation including microscopic evaluation for infectious agents, allergy testing, and even a colonoscopy. By clearly defining the past history of diarrhea, duration of episodes, and frequency of occurrence, the most appropriate evaluation can be undertaken.

Your differential diagnosis may be drawn more to an infectious etiology if you ascertain that the patient has recently been to a picnic where food may have been left out, eaten undercooked foods, or traveled to areas with unsanitary water supplies.

It is also important to ask about other family members or contacts with similar conditions. It should be noted if patients have recently dined out. If a community outbreak should occur, this information will be invaluable in the contribution to isolating the infectious cause.

BQ: A recent course of antibiotics may suggest *Clostridium difficile* as the infectious agent. Recently eating fried rice may suggest *Bacillus cereus*.

One should also discern the presence of excessive flatulence, explosive qualities and the presence of blood or mucous in the stools.

Within the symptoms associated, it is important to ask about fever, chills, nausea, and vomiting. If vomiting is present, it is again important to ask about frequency and last occurrence. Is the patient able to tolerate liquids? Severe vomiting and diarrhea may quickly lead to dehydration and electrolyte disturbances and require aggressive intervention.

Congratulations! You have completed the history section and soon you will start to learn the examination component. I'm sure you are excited to know that we will come back to more history taking when we come to the comprehensive Flows.

PHYSICAL EXAMINATION FLOWS

4

This chapter introduces you to the physical examination (PE). It is based on a systems approach. I like to approach the body from head to toe, and from front to back. These Flows are best practiced in groups of two to three. If you have two people in your group, one becomes the provider and the second the patient, who also checks off the Flow Sheet when a specific part of the examination is completed. If you have the ability to have three people, then the third person can evaluate the technique of examination and check off the areas of examination when each is completed. This allows for less interruption by the patient who will not have to check off each section of the Flow as it is completed, as in the prior scenario.

If you are using this text in association with a class, you should familiarize yourself with the Flow prior to the class session so that you will recognize the components of the Flow as they are presented.

Just like the history, the PE begins prior to your entering the room.

True Story

When I was in residency, we were lucky enough to have a small conference room in our primary care clinic that had large windows overlooking the parking lot. As I was finishing my charting late in the day, a small car came flying into the parking lot. A young lady jumped out of the car and literally ran into the building. I guessed that she was my last patient, who as almost a half hour late. The appointment list didn't say what she was coming in for and I hadn't recognized her or her name.

I was training students at the time, and typically would send one in to see the patient first so that they could develop their history taking skills. But this time, after about 20 minutes the student returned rather dismayed. The patient's chief complaint was back pain following an accident. The student was unable to examine her well because she could not lift herself off of the table for the examination. Was this the same women who I had observed jumping out of her car and running into the building? Sure enough, when we entered the room, there she was, lying on the table, barely able to move.

I probed her history again, adding to what the student had presented to me. About 3 weeks earlier, the patient was in her apartment when a water-soaked ceiling tile fell and hit her in the head. She now had neck and back pain. When I asked her if she had sought medical attention before now, she professed that she hadn't. I further discovered that she was able to seek out an attorney earlier in the day and was planning to file a suit. I was able to perform a complete examination with a little coaxing, and treated the patient conservatively as she lacked signs of serious injury. I advised her to come back in 1 week if she did not improve. After escorting her out of the room, my student and I dashed back to the conference room to witness her departure. Minutes later, this same young lady—who could barely get up off the exam table—dashed out of the front door of our building, and literally ran to her car, dove into the front seat, and squealed out of the parking lot. All of this was documented in her chart. Sure enough, 1 week to the day, she returned for persistent pain. I did not get the chance to see her in the parking lot, but while in the exam room she was barely able to sit up on the exam table. I updated her history and again completed a detailed examination. At this point, it was time to let the cat out of the bag. I explained to her that I had seen her both arrive and depart from her last office visit. I witnessed her running into and out of the office, and had documented what I had seen in her chart. I found her examination and ability to run to be incompatible with the professed disability in the examination room. I doubted her attorney would find my records constructive; however, because her pain persisted, I did order radiographs. I don't have an ending to this story as after she left my office that day, she never came back.

So you see, my examination began before I went into her room. Thousands of dollars of resources could have been spent on this fabricated complaint in the pursuit of X-rays, MRIs, physical therapy, and medications.

The PE Flows begin with a general assessment and vital signs and essentially moves cephalocaudal. You do not have to follow the system order as it is presented, but the important thing is to do your exam in the same way each time so that you do not skip an area. Again, you should not memorize the Flows; they should be approached logically.

The order of examination begins with inspection. Unless you are visually impaired, the first thing you do when entering the room is look at the patient, and then you touch or palpate. The next technique is percussion, followed by auscultation. Therefore, the order of examination is: Inspection, Palpation, Percussion and Auscultation (IPPA). Of course, there has to be an exception and that would be the abdomen where auscultation occurs immediately after inspection. This is logical in that palpation prior to auscultation would change the bowel sounds.

Here are several examples to clarify what is meant by "head to toe and front to back." When you perform the HEENT (Head, Ears, Eyes, Nose, Throat) Flow, the first thing you encounter at the top is the hair: inspect and palpate it. The next thing you encounter is the scalp: inspect and palpate it. Moving further downward is the skull where we can see boney deformity and then palpate. I examine the ears laterally, then, moving to the front, I see the forehead and face in general. Next, I encounter the eyes, nose and mouth, and so on, always moving downward. In my mind this is a logical progression. You should develop a pattern of exam for yourself that is logical to you so that when you complete an examination of one area, you drift easily into the next.

When you approach the ear, you look at the external ear first, examining all the skin areas including behind the ears where basal cell carcinomas like to hide. Then you work your way inward, past the conchal bowls, the cups around the external canal. Then you follow the canal until you see the tympanic membrane and finally, you visualize what you can behind the membrane, like boney prominences or fluid. You have gone front to back.

If you approach each body area this way, you will miss very little. Don't forget to test function. You just examined the entire ear but how does it hear? You can test function either before inspection or after auscultation. I would not interject it between IPPA because you will likely get lost. If you do get lost, just revert back to IPPA. "I've inspected and palpated. Oh yeah, now I have to percuss."

Not all body areas will need each component of IPPA. For example, there is no percussion in the heart flow.

I would highly recommend a good history and physical examination textbook to go along with this workbook. When an area of examination seems confusing, referencing the text will clarify proper technique.

① _____
Stacey = safer
austlaw = lander

② _____
_____

GENERAL ASSESSMENT AND VITAL SIGNS FLOW

Flow #1

		Performed
I.	INTRODUCES SELF	1
II.	EXPLAINS that physical exam will now be performed.	2
III.	GENERAL ASSESSMENT	
	A. Nutritional status—well nourished, malnourished, obese	3
	B. Level of consciousness—alert, lethargic, obtunded, stuporous	4
	C. Distress—respiratory, cardiac, pain, anxiety	5
	D. Development	6
	E. Skin coloration—pallor, cyanosis, jaundice	7
	F. Hygiene—unkempt, malodor, well groomed	8
	G. Posture/position of comfort	9
IV.	VITALS	
	A. TEMPERATURE—NORMAL VALUES	
	1. Rectal—one degree above oral	10
	2. Oral	11
	3. Axillary—one degree below oral	12
	B. PULSE	
	1. Calculate rate—measure for 15 seconds and multiply by 4	13
	2. Note rhythm	14
	3. Note character	15
	C. RESPIRATIONS	
	1. Check rate for a full minute	16
	2. Note rhythm	17
	3. Note character	18
	D. BLOOD PRESSURE	
	1. Have patient sit for 5 minutes	19
	2. Question patient about nicotine/caffeine in the last 30 minutes	20
	3. Bare arm	21
	4. Locate the brachial artery	22
	5. Apply cuff 2.5 cm proximal to antecubital fossa	23
	6. Assure the appropriate size cuff	24
	7. Inflate while palpating radial artery, note disappearance	25
	8. Deflate and reinflate to 20 mm Hg above disappearance	26
	9. Auscultate brachial artery	27
	10 Deflate cuff at a rate of 2–3 mm per second	28
	11. Note first sounds to return—systolic	29
	12. Note muffling point	30

GENERAL ASSESSMENT AND VITAL SIGNS FLOW

Flow #1

Performed

	13.	Note disappearance point—diastolic pressure	31
	14.	Repeat in other arm	32
E.		PAIN—Rate pain on a scale and describe scale to patient	33
III.		SPECIAL CONSIDERATIONS	
A.		Describe ausculatory gap	34
B.		Suspect blood volume loss or syncope	
	1.	Take in supine, seated and then standing positions	35
	2.	Define orthostatic hypotension: 20 mm Hg fall	36

NOTES:

INTEGUMENTARY FLOW

Flow #2

				Performed
I.	INTRODUCES SELF			1
II.	EXPLAINS that physical exam will now be performed.			2
III.	Educate the patient on the ABCDs of melanoma			
	A.	Asymmetry		3
	B.	Border irregularity		4
	C.	Color variation		5
	D.	Diameter greater than 6 mm		6
IV.	HAIR			
	A.	INSPECTION		
		1.	Scalp—patterns of loss	7
		2.	Eyebrows—lateral loss in hypothyroidism (myxedema)	8
		3.	Facial hair—maturity, hirsutism	9
		4.	Infestations	10
	B.	PALPATION—Texture		
		1.	Fine, oily, abundant in thyrotoxicosis	11
		2.	Dry, course, thinning with easy fragmentation in myxedema	12
V.	SKIN			
	A.	INSPECTION		
		1.	Appropriate exposure	13
		2.	Generalized scanning—symmetry, exposure, tendency toward lesions	14
		3.	Thickness	15
		4.	Color	
			a. Generalized uniformity	
			(1) Red (Erythema)—polycythemia, carbon monoxide, drug rxn, exanthem	16
			(2) White (Pallor)—albinism, anemia	17
			(3) Blue (Cyanosis)—hypoxia	18
			(4) Yellow (Jaundice)—hyperbilirubinemia, hemolysis, liver disease	19
			(5) Brown (Hyperpigmentation)—pituitary, adrenal or liver disfunction	20
			b. Localized discoloration	
			(1) Red—inflammation, hemangioma	21
			(2) White (Amelanotic)—vitiligo, scar	22
			(3) Blue—venous pooling, nevi	23
			(4) Brown—nevi, café au lait, melanoma	24

INTEGUMENTARY FLOW   Flow #2

                                                         Performed

B.		PALPATION		
	1.	Moisture		
		a.	Dry, moist, diaphoretic, oily	25
		b.	Examine skin folds	26
	2.	Temperature		
		a.	Cool, warm, hot	27
		b.	Palpation with back of hand comparing symmetrically	28
	3.	Texture—soft, rough, smooth, even		29
	4.	Turgor and mobility		
		a.	Pinch skin on forearm and release. Do not pinch dorsum of hand.	30
		b.	Delayed turgor = dehydration or edema	31
		c.	Decreased mobility—connective tissue disease	32
	5.	Lesions—define by:		
		a.	Size	33
		b.	Shape/configuration—ovoid, annular, linear, clustered, diffuse, confluent	34
		c.	Color	35
		d.	Type—macule, papule, patch, plaque, vesical, bulla, ulceration, nodule, cyst	36
		e.	Location	37
		f.	Border	38
C.		NAILS		
	1.	Hygiene—bitten, clean, manicured		39
	2.	Color—pink, cyanosis, yellowing (psoriasis), whitening, green (pseudomonas)		40
	3.	Clubbing—hypoxia, cirrhosis, thyroid disorder		41
	4.	Lesions—pigmentation (melanoma), splinter hemorrhages (endocarditis)		42
	5.	Nail folds—lesions (warts), inflammation		43
	6.	Capillary refill: > 2 seconds = hypoperfusion		44

NOTES:

HEENT FLOW (Head, Eyes, Ear, Nose, Throat)   Flow #3

Performed

I.	INTRODUCES SELF		1
II.	EXPLAINS that physical exam will now be performed.		2
III.	HEAD		
	A.	Inspection	
		1. Symmetry and form (normocephalic, microcephalic, macrocephalic)	3
		2. Hair (see Integumentary system)	4
		3. Scalp—lesions, rash	5
		4. Face—symmetry (cranial nerve seven) and lesions	6
	B.	Palpation: masses, boney deformity	7
IV.	EYES		
	A.	Function—visual acuity by hand chart or wall chart	8
	B.	Visual Fields	
	C.	Inspection	
		1. Position of the eye by light reflection—rule out strabismus	9
		2. Visible sclera above the iris—rule out exophthalmus	10
		3. Extraocular movements (cranial nerves III, IV, and VI)	11
		4. Cornea—clouding, lesions, injection	12
		5. Perpendicular light across iris—rule out shallow anterior chamber	13
		6. Pupil-size, shape, symmetry, reaction (direct and consensual)	14
		7. Sclera—injection, icterus, lesion, hemorrhage	15
		8. Conjunctiva—injection, pallor, foreign body (inverting upper lid), exudate	16
		9. Ophthalmoscopic examination	
		a. Identify the Cup and Disk—note ratio and papilledema	17
		b. Identify retinal deformities—detachment, lesions	18
		c. Identify vascular abnormalities—diabetic retinopathy, hypertensive changes	19
V.	EARS		
	A.	Function—auditory acuity by whispered word with contralateral occluded ear	20
	B.	If hearing loss is suspected discern between conductive and sensorineural hearing loss	21
		1. Rhinne test—compares air conduction (AC) with bone conduction (BC)	22
		a. Strike 512 Hz tuning fork and place handle on mastoid process	23
		b. Ask patient if sound can be heard, and if so, when it stops	24
		c. When sound stops, move tines in front of ear, and ask if patient can hear it again	25

HEENT FLOW (Head, Eyes, Ear, Nose, Throat) Flow #3

						Performed

					Performed
	d.	Interpretation			
		(1)	AC is better than (>) BC = Rhinne Positive = normal or sensorineural hearing loss with impaired air and bone conduction		26
		(2)	BC > AC = Rhinne Negative = conductive hearing loss		27
	2.	Weber test—compares bone conduction in each ear			28
		a.	Strike 512 Hz tuning fork, place handle on the center of patient's forehead		29
		b.	Ask patient which ear sound is heard or felt best: in right, left, or equally		30
		c.	Interpretation		
			(1)	Sound is heard or felt midline = normal test, no conductive loss	31
			(2)	Sound is heard toward one side = lateralization	32
				(a) To affected side in conductive loss	33
				sounds louder due to absence of background noise	
				(b) To unaffected side in sensorineural loss	34
C.	Inspection				
	1.	External ear: deformity, lesions			35
	2.	External canal exudate			36
	3.	Palpate tragus and pinna prior to insertion of otoscope for pain differentiates otitis externa from otitis media			37
	4.	Otoscopic examination			
		a.	Position canal: retract pinna up, out, and back for adult down, out, and back for child		38 / 39
		b.	Insert otoscope with inverted hold, distending 5th digit		40
		c.	Examine canal for lesions, exudate, errythema, cerumen		41
		d.	Inspect tympanic membrane: color, light reflex, boney structure		42
		e.	Identify perforation, bulging or retraction		43
		f.	Insuffilate for mobility of tympanic membrane		44
VI. NOSE					
	A.	Inspection			
		1.	External surface for deformity, lesions		45
		2.	Nares—for exudate and symmetry		46
		3.	Otoscopic examination		
			a.	Have patient tilt the head back	47

HEENT FLOW (Head, Eyes, Ear, Nose, Throat)

Flow #3

Performed

	b.	Inspect for lesion, foreign bodies, epistaxis, discharge, polyps	48
	c.	Identify septum (perforation, deviation), turbinates	49
B.		Palpation—check for nasal patency by occluding nare and having patient breathe in	50

VII. SINUSES

A.	Inspection—transilluminate the frontal, maxillary, and ethmoid sinuses	51
B.	Percussion and Palpation—for tenderness	52

VIII. THROAT

A.	Inspection		
	1.	Lips for lesions, fissures, color (pallor, cyanosis)	53
	2.	Buccal mucosa	
		a.　Lesions	54
		b.　Stenson ducts orifice—parotid gland opening adjacent to 2nd upper molar	55
		c.　Gingiva—retraction, bleeding, hypertrophy, swelling	56
	3.	Teeth—state of repair, erosions, broken teeth, caries	57
	4.	Roof of mouth—hard and soft palate for lesions, clefts	58
	5.	Tongue—lesions	59
	6.	Floor of mouth—lesions, Wharton duct (opening of the submandibular gland)	60
	7.	Tonsillar pillars and tonsils if present	61
	8.	Posterior pharynx	
		a.　Have patient phonate—identify lesions, discharge	62
		b.　Use a tongue blade if necessary, avoiding the gag reflex	63
B.	Palpation with gloves		
	1.	Lips and buccal mucosa	64
	2.	Parotid gland	65
	3.	Tongue and floor of mouth	66

NOTES:

NECK AND LYMPHATICS FLOW

Flow #4

			Performed
I.	INTRODUCES SELF		1
II.	EXPLAINS that physical exam will now be performed.		2
III.	NECK		
	A. Inspection		
		1. Symmetry	3
		2. Lesions	4
		3. Masses	5
		4. Tracheal position	6
		5. Jugular venous distension	7
	B. Range of motion (ROM)—(see musculoskeletal flow)		
	C. Auscultation prior to palpation		8
		1. Carotids—for bruit	9
		2. Thyroid—for bruit	10
	D. Palpation		
		1. Posterior anatomy—with provider in front of seated or at head of supine patient	
		a. Nuchal cord—rigidity	11
		b. Cervical spinous processes	12
		c. Paravertebral musculature/transverse processes	13
		2. Anterior—with provider behind seated patient	
		a. Cricoid and thyroid cartilage	14
		b. Position of trachea	15
		c. Thyroid—have patient swallow—for nodules, thyroidmegaly	16
		d. Carotids—detract sternocleidomastoid posteriorly with pads of two fingers	17
IV.	LYMPHATICS		
	A. Cervical		
		1. Inspection—visible lymphadenopathy	18
		2. Palpation—note size, mobility, tenderness	19
		a. Anterior auricular	20
		b. Posterior auricular	21
		c. Submental	22
		d. Submandibular	23
		e. Posterior cervical chain	24
		f. Anterior cervical chain	25

NECK AND LYMPHATICS FLOW	Flow #4
	Performed
g. Supraclavicular	26
h. Infraclavicular	27
B. Axillary	
1. Position patient in seated position with arms at side	28
2. Palpation	29
C. Extremities	
1. Areas—inguinal, epitrochlear	30
2. Inspection—visible lymphadenopathy	31
3. Palpation—lymphadenopathy	32
V. Suspected Meningitis	
A. Nuchal rigidity	33
B. Brudzinski—patient supine, passively flex neck (+ sign = pain or restricted flexion)	34
C. Kernig—patient supine, knees bent, extend lower leg (+ sign = pain)	35

NOTES:

RESPIRATORY FLOW

Flow #5

		Performed
I.	INTRODUCES SELF	1
II.	EXPLAINS that physical exam will now be performed.	2
III.	INSPECTION	
	A. Appropriately expose the chest	3
	B. Assess for signs of respiratory distress	
	1. Cyanosis	4
	2. Accessory muscle use	5
	3. Intercostal retractions	6
	4. Nasal flaring	7
	C. Assess rate and rhythm	8
	D. Note position of comfort: tripod, leaning forward, head of bed elevated	9
	E. Skin	
	1. Color: cyanosis (blue blower), pallor, erythema (pink puffer), cherry red	10
	2. Nails: clubbing	11
	F. Eyes: conjunctival pallor	12
	G. Neck: position of trachea	13
	H. Chest	
	1. Wall symmetry with rise and fall	14
	2. Deformity: pectus excavatum, pectus carinatum, boney deformity, flail chest	15
	3. Anterior/Posterior: Lateral ratio (AP:lat ratio), barrel chest	16
IV.	PALPATION	
	A. Soft tissues: tenderness	17
	B. Deep structures: boney deformity, reproducible pain	18
	C. Symmetrical expansion: anterior and posterior	19
	D. Tactile fremitus: uses medial hand margin, symmetrical approach	20
	E. Rib dysfunction: resistance to inspiration or expiration	21
V.	PERCUSSION	
	A. Symmetrical approach for each level, anterior, posterior, and lateral	22
	B. Diaphragmatic excursion	23
VI.	AUSCULTATION	
	A. Instructs patient to take deep breaths, slowly, through the mouth	24
	B. Auscultates through complete inspiration and expiration	25
	C. Symmetrically	
	1. Anteriorly: three levels including supraclavicular	26
	2. Posteriorly: minimum of three levels	27
	3. Laterally	28

RESPIRATORY FLOW	Flow #5
	Performed

	D.	Identify adventitious sounds—crackles, rhonchi, wheezes, rubs	29
VII.	SPECIAL TESTING if suspecting consolidation		
	A.	Bronchophony: sound transmitted louder at area of consolidation	30
	B.	Egophony: patient says "e", sounds like "a" at areas of consolidation	31
	C.	Whispered pectoriloquy: whispered word sounds louder at area of consolidation	32
VIII.	CLINICAL SCENARIOS: expected findings for tactile fremitus and percussion for each		
	A.	Pneumonia: increased tactile fremitus, decreased resonance on percussion	33
	B.	Pneumothorax: decreased tactile fremitus, increased resonance on percussion	34
	C.	Pleural effusion: decreased tactile fremitus, decreased resonance on percussion	35

NOTES:

w/ pneumonia = ↑ tactile fremitus , ↓ percussion (dull)
consolidation

↓ pneumothorax = ↓ tactile fremitus ; ↑ percussion
(hypertympanic)

pleural effusion = ↓ tactile fremitus = ↓ percussion (dull)

CARDIOVASCULAR FLOW

Handwritten: Vital Sign) (2arms → 2bps)
[? if syncope = ortho...] ?

Flow #6

Performed

I.	**INTRODUCES SELF**		1
II.	**EXPLAINS** that physical exam will now be performed.		2
III.	**EYES**: ophthalmoscopic examination for hypertensive retinopathy		3
IV.	**NECK**		
	A.	Inspect for JVD (measure centimeters of elevation and degree recumbency)	4
	B.	Auscultate for bruits prior to palpation in the elderly	5
	C.	Palpate the carotids separately	6
V.	**CHEST**		
	A.	Inspection	
		1. Stand on right side of patient and examine precordial area with tangental lighting	7
		2. Visualize: PMI, heaves	8
	B.	Identify cardiac areas of palpation and auscultation	
		1. Aortic: 2nd right intercostal space (ICS) along sternal border	9
		2. Pulmonic: 2nd left intercostal space along sternal border	10
		3. Tricuspid: 4th or 5th left intercostal space along sternal border	11
		4. Mitral: 4th or 5th intercostal space mid-clavicular line	12
	C.	Palpation	
		1. Thrills using metacarpal phalangeal joints	13
		2. Point of maximal impulse (PMI)—use pad of finger: note ICS and vertical location	14
	D.	Auscultation	
		1. Note rate and rhythm	15
		2. Note character of first (S1) and second heart sound (S2)	
		a. S1—closure of AV valves (marks onset of systole)	16
		b. S2—closure of the semilunar valves (aortic, pulmonic)	17
		3. Assess splitting of S2—r side slightly delayed with decreased pressures (A2>P2)	18
		a. Have patient exhale and hold (resolves physiologic split, not IHSS)	19
	E.	Extra Sounds *(= HOCM)*	
		1. Ejection click—early systole = diseased aortic valve	20
		2. Opening snap—early diastole = mitral disease	21
		3. S3 = rapid deceleration of blood. Decreased compliance in adults.	22
		4. S4 = atrial kick against decreased compliance.	23
	F.	Murmurs	
		1. Timing (systolic, diastolic) and duration (early, middle, late, or pan)	24

CARDIOVASCULAR FLOW

Flow #6

Performed

	2.	Shape		
		a.	Crescendo/decrescendo—aortic stenosis	25
		b.	Plateau—mitral regurgitation, tricuspid regurg, ventriculoseptal defect	26
		c.	Decrescendo—aortic regurgitation	27
	3.	Location—valvular area		28
	4.	Radiation—neck (aortic stenosis), axilla (mitral regurgitation)		29
	5.	Intensity—discuss grades 1 through 6[1]		
			Grade 1—Very faint, possibly not heard in all positions	30
			Grade 2—Easily heard but faint	31
			Grade 3—Moderately loud	32
			Grade 4—Loud with palpable thrill	33
			Grade 5—Heard with stethoscope partially off of the chest	34
			Grade 6—Heard with stethoscope off the chest	35
	6.	Pitch (low, medium, or high)		36
	7.	Quality (musical, rumbling, blowing, harsh)		37
G.	Special Positions			
	1.	Left lateral decubitus (mitral stenosis, S3, S4)		38
	2.	Sitting, leaning forward, breathe out and hold (aortic murmur)		39
	3.	Standing, squatting, valsalva (MVP and aortic stenosis)		40
VI.	ABDOMEN			
A.	Auscultation: aorta, renal, iliac, and femoral artery bruits			41
B.	Palpation			
	1.	Size of aorta for aneurysm		42
	2.	Hepatojugular reflex		43
V.	EXTREMITIES			
A.	Inspection			
	1.	Edema—scale 0–4 (1 = ankle, 2 = tibia, 3 = femoral, 4 = sacrum)		44
	2.	Varicosities		45
	3.	Stasis dermatitis pigmentation and ulcerations (valvular incompetency)		46
	4.	Hair loss (peripheral arterial disease)		47
	5.	Nail beds (splinter hemorrhages with endocarditis)		48
B.	Palpation			
	1.	Compare b/l brachial, radial, femoral, popliteal, dorsalis pedis, post tibialis		49
	2.	Capillary refill—normal refill is less than 3 seconds		50
	3.	Signs of phlebitis—venous tenderness, cords, warmth		51

CARDIOVASCULAR FLOW

Flow #6

			Performed
C.	Allen Test—define test as competency of radial and ulnar arteries		52
	1.	Palm up	53
	2.	Have patient clench fist	54
	3.	Compress radial and ulnar artery	55
	4.	Have patient relax hand	56
	5.	Observe pale palm	57
	6.	Release ulnar artery	58
	7.	Findings	
		a. Normal = pinks in 3–5 seconds	59
		b. Abnormal—repeat releasing radial artery	60

NOTES:

NOTES:

ABDOMINAL FLOW

Flow #7

Performed

I.	INTRODUCES SELF		1
II.	EXPLAINS that the physical exam will now be performed.		2
III.	INSPECTION		
	A.	Properly expose the abdomen	3
	B.	Provider standing on right side of supine patient	4
	C.	General contour of abdomen—flat, scaphoid, distended	5
	D.	Asymmetry, masses	6
	E.	Lesions, scars	7
	F.	Umbilucus, venous pattern (caput medusa)	8
	G.	Have patient flex forward—assess for hernias, rectus diathesis	9
VI.	AUSCULATION		
	A.	Prior to percussion and palpation	10
	B.	Four quadrants	11
	C.	Identify bowel sounds—normoactive, hypoactive, and hyperactive	12
	D.	Characterize bowel sounds—tinkling, borborigomi	13
	E.	Arterial bruits—(see Cardiovascular Flow #6)	14
V.	PALPATION		
	A.	Watches facial expression for grimace during palpation	15
	B.	Begins in quadrant furthest from complaint of pain if present	16
	C.	If abdomen is too tense, have patient bend knees placing feet flat on the table	17
	D.	Light palpation assessing skin and subcutaneous tissues using finger pads of one hand	18
		1. Tenderness	19
		2. Masses	20
	E.	Deep palpation assessing visceral structures using one hand on top the other	21
		1. Tenderness	22
		2. Masses	23
		3. Hepatomegaly—begin in RLQ and roll fingers upward to the R costal margin	24
		4. Splenomegaly—begin at umbilicus rolling fingers diagonally to the L costal margin	25
		5. Uterine height	26
		6. Bladder distension	27
		7. Size of aorta	28

ABDOMINAL FLOW

Flow #7

Performed

VI.	PERCUSSION	
	A. Assess pattern of resonance—hyperresonant, dull, gastric bubble	29
	B. Liver span	30
VII.	CLINICAL SCENARIOS	
	A. Acute abdomen	
	1. Assess for guarding, rigidity, rebound (ask patient which hurts more, pushing in: push in slowly but deeply; or letting go: suddenly lift hand from depressed position)	31
	2. Rovsing sign—pain in RLQ with LLQ pressure	32
	3. Psoas sign—flexion and extension of hip	33
	4. Obturator sign—flex hip and internally rotate	34
	5. Rectal exam	35
	6. Vaginal exam	36
	B. Ascities	
	1. Shifting dullness	37
	2. Fluid wave	38
	C. Cholecystitis—Murphy sign: push up under RCM, have patient take a deep breath in. Suddenly halting breath is a + sign.	39
	D. Neprolithiasis, hydronephrosis, pyelonephritis—CVA tenderness (Lloyds punch)	40

NOTES:

MUSCULOSKELETAL FLOW

Flow #8

Performed

I.	INTRODUCES SELF	1
II.	EXPLAINS that the physical exam will now be performed.	2
III.	GENERAL INSPECTION	
	A. Body symmetry: compare bilateral upper and lower extremity muscle mass	3
	B. Head: normocephalic, microcephalic, hydrocephalic, syndromal appearance	4
	C. Identify limb or boney deformity	5
	D. Compares all joint exams bilaterally	6
IV.	TEMPOROMANDIBULAR JOINT (TMJ)	
	A. Visualize active ROM—assure midline movement	7
	B. Palpation—place pad of index finger in conchal bowl, identify clicking	8
V.	SHOULDERS	
	A. Inspect for symmetry, boney deformity	9
	B. Active range of motion (AROM)—abduction, adduction, flexion, extension	10
	C. Passive ROM if limited in AROM	11
	D. Palpation	
	1. Joint structure—sternoclavicular, clavicle, acromioclavicular	12
	2. Rotator cuff	13
	3. Bicipital groove with elbow bent at 90 degrees and external rotation	14
VI.	ELBOWS	
	A. Inspect for symmetry, boney deformity	15
	B. AROM—flexion, extension, supination, pronation	16
	C. Passive ROM if limited in AROM	17
	D. Palpation	
	1. Joint structure—olecranon, epicondyles	18
	2. Bursa—olecranon	19
VII.	WRISTS	
	A. Inspect for symmetry, boney deformity	20
	B. AROM—abduction, adduction, flexion, extension	21
	C. Passive ROM if limited in AROM	22
	D. Palpation—including anatomical snuff box (indicator of scaphoid fracture)	23
VIII.	FINGERS	
	A. Inspect for symmetry, boney deformity	
	1. Heberden nodes—distal interphalangeal joint—osteoarthritis	24
	2. Bouchard nodes—proximal interphalangeal joint—rheumatoid arthritis	25
	B. AROM—abduction, adduction, flexion, extension	26
	C. Passive ROM if limited in AROM	27

MUSCULOSKELETAL FLOW

Flow #8

Performed

IX.	HIPS		
	A.	Inspect for symmetry, boney deformity	28
	B.	AROM—abduction, adduction, flexion, extension, internal and external rotation	29
	C.	Passive ROM if limited in AROM	30
	D.	Bursa: greater trochanteric	31
X.	KNEES		
	A.	Inspect for symmetry, boney deformity, varus or valgus deviation (standing position)	32
	B.	AROM—flexion and extension	33
	C.	Passive ROM if limited in AROM	34
	D.	Palpation	
		1. Popliteal fossa with patient standing—Baker cyst	35
		2. Peripatellar	36
		3. Medial and lateral joint spaces	37
		4. Tibial tubercle	38
XI.	ANKLES/FEET		
	A.	Inspect for symmetry, boney deformity, pes planus (in standing position)	39
	B.	AROM—dorsiflexion, plantarflexion, inversion, eversion, internal and external rotation	40
	C.	Passive ROM if limited in AROM	41
	D.	Palpation: medial and lateral malleoli, deltoid ligament, Achilles tendon	42
XII.	SPINE		
	A.	Inspection	
		1. From side—note changes in lordosis and kyphosis	43
		2. From behind—note rotoscoliosis (lateral curvature)	44
	B.	AROM—flexion, extension, rotation, sidebending stabilizing patient at hips	45
	C.	Passive ROM if limited in AROM	46
	D.	Palpation: spinous and transverse processes, paravertebral musculature	47
XIII.	CLINICAL SCENARIOS		
	A.	Knee injury	
		1. Ballottement—fluid in joint space	48
		2. Varus and valgus stress—collateral ligament stability	49
		3. Anterior drawer—anterior cruciate ligament (ACL) stability	50
		4. Posterior drawer—posterior cruciate ligament (PCL) stability	51
		5. McMurray sign and Apley grind—Meniscal tear	52

MUSCULOSKELETAL FLOW

Flow #8

Performed

B.   Back pain

    1.   Straight leg raise—patient supine, providers hands under heals of patient   53

    2.   Seated straight leg raise—if suspicion of factitious disorder   54

C.   Carpal tunnel

    1.   Phalen sign

            55

    2.   Tinel sign

            56

NOTES:

NOTES:

OSTEOPATHIC MANIPULATIVE MEDICINE FLOW

Flow #9

Performed

I.	INTRODUCES SELF		1
II.	EXPLAINS that the physical examination is about to be performed.		2
III.	SEATED		
	A.	Inspection—symmetry	3
	B.	Seated flexion test	4
IV.	STANDING		
	A.	Inspection—symmetry	
		1. Earlobes	5
		2. Shoulders	6
		3. Inferior scapula	7
		4. Iliac crests	8
		5. Ischial tuberosities	9
	B.	Palpation—in neutral position	
		1. Spinal curvature—thoracic, lumbar	
		a. Spinous processes	10
		b. Transverse processes	11
		2. ROM	
		a. Thoracic sidebending	
		(1) T1.	12
		(2) T4	13
		(3) T10	14
		3. Standing flexion test	15
		4. Repeat in flexion	16
		5. Repeat in extension	17
V.	PRONE		
	A.	Inspection—symmetry	
		1. Medial malleoli	18
		2. Ischial tuberosities	19
		3. Iliac crests	20
		4. Inferior scapula	21
	B.	Palpation	
		1. Spinal curvature—thoracic, lumbar	
		a. Spinous processes	22
		b. Transverse processes	23

OSTEOPATHIC MANIPULATIVE MEDICINE FLOW

Flow #9

Performed

	2.	Sacrum		
		a.	Sacroiliac joint	24
		b.	Sacral sulci	25
		c.	Inferior lateral angles (ILAs)	26
	3.	Ischial tuberosities		27
	4.	Spring test		28
VI.	SUPINE			
	A.	Inspection—symmetry		
		1.	Medial malleoli	29
		2.	Iliac crests	30
		3.	First rib	31
	B.	ROM		
		1.	L5	32
		2.	T12.	33
		3.	First rib	34
		4.	C7	35
		5.	C4	36
		6.	C1.	37
	C.	Translation—cervical		38
	D.	Palpation		
		1.	Cervical	
			a. Spinous processes	39
			b. Transverse processes	40
			c. OA	41
		2.	Cranial rhythmic impulse	42

NOTES:

NEUROLOGICAL FLOW

Flow #10

	Performed

I. INTRODUCES SELF — 1

II. EXPLAINS that the physical exam will now be performed. — 2

III. RESPONSIVENESS: alert, lethargic, responds to verbal stimulation, touch or pain, comatose — 3

IV. ORIENTATION: person, place, time — 4

V. GENERAL ASSESSMENT: posture, obvious extremity weakness or asymmetry — 5

VI. CRANIAL NERVE (CN) EXAMINATION[2]

  A. Memory trigger: On Old Olympus' Towering Tops A Finn And German Viewed Some Hops — 6

  B. CNI—Olfactory — 7

    1. Have patient close the eyes and occlude one nare. Place source of smell under open nare and have patient identify it. — 8

    2. Repeat with second source for other nare. — 9

  C. CNII—Optic — 10

    1. Assess visual acuity — 11

    2. Assess peripheral fields — 12

    3. Memory trigger for pupillary reflex: In by 2 out by 3 — 13

    4. Pupillary reflex: direct and consensual (sensory component of pupillary reflex) — 14

  D. CNIII—Occulomotor — 15

    1. Pupillary reflex: direct and consensual (motor component of pupillary reflex) — 16

    2. Memory trigger: extraocular movements (EOM) LR6 SO4 Remainder 3 — 17

    3. Extraocular movements

      a. Medial rectus—moves eyes medially (accommodation) — 18

      b. Inferior oblique—moves eyes upward and inward — 19

      c. Superior rectus—moves eyes upward and laterally — 20

      d. Inferior rectus—moves eyes downward and laterally — 21

    4. Ptosis: upper lid is held up by the pillar III — 22

  E. CNIV—Trochlear: EOM: superior oblique (moves eyes down and inward) — 23

  F. CNV—Trigeminal — 24

    1. Motor branch—have patient clench the teeth, palpating muscles of mastication — 25

    2. Sensory branch—test sensation in each branch of the trigeminal — 26

    3. Corneal reflex—touch cornea with strand of cotton ball with lateral approach — 27

  G. CNVI—Abducens: EOM lateral rectus (moves eyes laterally) — 28

NEUROLOGICAL FLOW

Flow #10

			Performed
H.	CNVII—Facial		29
	1.	Motor branch	
		a. Facial symmetry—raise eyebrows, frown, smile, puff cheeks, show teeth	30
		b. Close eyes: memory trigger—think of "7" as a hook pulling the eyelid down	31
	2.	Sensory branch—test for taste in anterior two thirds of tongue	32
I.	CNVIII—Acoustic (vestibulocochlear)		33
	1.	Test hearing—whispered word (see HEENT Flow for deficiency testing)	34
	2.	Vestibular function—assess for nystagmus	35
J.	CNIX—Glossopharyngeal		36
	1.	Have patient open mouth and say "ahh" assessing for symmetrical rise of uvula	37
	2.	Identify deviation of uvula as away from side of neurologic lesion	38
	3.	Sensory component of gag reflex: posterior tongue and pharynx	39
	4.	Taste to posterior one third of tongue	40
K.	CNX—Vagus		41
	1.	Motor component of gag reflex	42
	2.	Assess for dysphonia—innervates the larynx	43
L.	CNXI—Spinal Accessory: motor		44
	1.	Have patient rotate head from 90 degrees to midline—sternocleidomastoid	45
	2.	Have patient shrug shoulders—trapezius	46
M.	CNXII—Hypoglossal		47
	1.	Observe tongue for fasciculations	48
	2.	Have patient stick the tongue outward	49
	3.	Identify deviation of tongue toward side of neurologic lesion	50
VII. MOTOR			
A.	Inspection for involuntary movements and muscle atrophy		51
B.	Strength Testing[3]		
	1.	Identify Scale as 0 to 5	
		a. 0 = no muscle twitch with attempted movement of muscle group	52
		b. 1 = twitch only of muscle with attempted movement	53
		c. 2 = movement against horizontal plane only, not against gravity	54
		d. 3 = movement against gravity but not against resistance	55
		e. 4 = movement against gravity and some resistance	56
		f. 5 = movement against full resistance	57

NEUROLOGICAL FLOW

Flow #10

Performed

2. Bilateral comparison

a.	Shoulder abduction—axillary nerve C5-6	58
b.	Elbow flexion—musculocutaneous nerve C5-6	59
c.	Elbow extension—radial nerve C6-8	60
d.	Wrist flexion—median nerve C6-7	61
e.	Wrist extension—radial nerve C6-8	62
f.	Grip—finger adduction—median nerve C6-8	63
g.	Finger abduction—ulnar nerve—C8-T1.	64
h.	Thumb abduction—median nerve C8-T1.	65
j.	Hip adduction—obturator nerve L2-4	66
k.	Hip abduction—superior gluteal nerve L4-S1.	67
l.	Knee extension—femoral nerve—L2-4	68
m.	Knee flexion—sciatic nerve L4-S1.	69
n.	Dorsiflexion—deep peroneal L4-5	70
o.	Plantarflexion—tibial L5-S2.	71

VIII. SENSORY

A. Symmetrical comparison throughout — 72

B. Techniques

1. Light touch—cotton wisp — 73
2. Sharp versus dull comparison—dispose of object used to test — 74
3. Temperature — 75
4. Vibration—using 128-Hz tuning fork — 76
5. Proprioception — 77
6. Discrimination

   a. Point localization—patient points to area touched — 78
   b. Extinction—asking patient if being touched on right side, left side or both — 79
   c. Two point distinction—may use paperclip adjusting width — 80
   d. Stereognosis—recognition of familiar object in palm with eyes closed — 81
   e. Graphesthesia—recognition of numbers drawn on palm with eyes closed — 83

IX. REFLEXES[4]

A. Identify scale as 0 to 4

1. 0 = no response — 84
2. 1 = diminished but present reflex — 85

| NEUROLOGICAL FLOW | Flow #10 |
| | Performed |

				Performed
		3.	2 = normal reflex	86
		4.	3 = somewhat increased reflex	87
		5.	4 = greatly increased reflex	88
	B.		Identify motor neuron disease	
		1.	Hyporeflexia suggests lower motor neuron disease	89
		2.	Hyperreflexia suggest upper motor neuron disease	90
	C.		Bilateral comparison	
		1.	Biceps: C5-6	91
		2.	Brachioradialis: C5-6	92
		3.	Triceps: C6-7	93
		4.	Patellar: L2-4	94
		5.	Achilles: S1-2.	95
	D.		Babinski sign: stroke lateral plantar surface of foot and cross medially at the ball	
		1.	Normal: first digit plantarflexes	96
		2.	Abnormal: first digit dorsiflexes—indicates upper motor neuron disease	97
X.			CEREBELLAR FUNCTION	
	A.		Rapid alternating movements	98
	B.		Finger to nose testing	99
	C.		Pronator drift—arms forward, palms up, close eyes	100
	D.		Heal to shin	101
	E.		Gait	102
	F.		Tandem walk—heel to toe	103
	G.		Romberg—feet together, arms out, palms up, close eyes	104
XI.			CLINICAL SCENARIOS	
	A.		Meningitis	
		1.	Neck mobility and nuchal rigidity	105
		2.	Brudzinski—supine, flex neck forward cause pain	106
		3.	Kerning—supine, flex patient's hip and knee, straighten knee causes pain	107
	B.		Dementia	
		1.	Perform mini mental status examination	108
		2.	Have patient draw the face of a clock	109

NOTES:

BREAST FLOW

Flow #11

Performed

I.	INTRODUCES SELF	1
II.	EXPLAINS that physical exam will now be performed.	2
III.	ENSURE that a female attendant is in the room if performing exam on a female	3
IV.	PATIENT EDUCATION	
	A. Advise breast self-examination (BSE) should be performed monthly.	4
	B. Discuss best time of month to perform (1 to 2 weeks after menses)	5
	C. Educate the patient on five clinical signs to watch for:	
	1. Change in nipple direction	6
	2. Masses	7
	3. Tenderness	8
	4. Dimpling of the skin	9
	5. Discharge	10
	D. Advise male patient: onset is usually in the 50s and located behind the nipple	11
V.	INSPECTION	
	A. Have patient seated on exam table with arms at side	12
	B. Expose both breasts to compare bilaterally	13
	C. Note Sexual Maturity Rating[5]	
	1. Stage 1 Elevation of nipple only	14
	2. Stage 2 Elevation of breast bud and areola	15
	3. Stage 3 Continued enlargement of breast and darkening of areola	16
	4. Stage 4 Areola rises as second mound. Contour change is noted.	17
	5. Stage 5 Mature breast—secondary mound blends back into single contour	18
	D. Examine for:	
	1. Changes in skin or coloration, lesions, texture, or dimpling	19
	2. Nipple deviation or retraction	20
	3. Asymmetry	21
	4. Gynecomastia in males	22
	E. Repeat examination with hands over head, and with hands on hips, leaning forward	23
VI.	PALPATION	
	A. Have patient in the supine position	24
	B. Cover breast that is not being examined	25
	C. Place rolled towel or pillow behind the shoulder and raise arm on the same side	26
	D. Palpate with pads of fingers with systematic approach (circles, linear)	27

BREAST FLOW

Flow #11

			Performed
E.		Palpate from midsternum to axilla and from inferior margin of breast to clavicle	28
F.		Gently squeeze nipple and note discharge	29
G.		Lymphatics	
	1.	Supraclavicular	30
	2.	Infraclavicular	31
	3.	Axillary: exam with patient's arm at side and elbow flexed	32
H.		Note consistency, nodules, and tenderness.	33

NOTES:

FEMALE GENITALIA AND RECTUM FLOW

Flow #12

		Performed
I.	INTRODUCES SELF	1
II.	EXPLAINS that physical exam will now be performed.	2
III.	PREPARATION	
	A. Ensure that a female attendant is in the room	3
	B. Position patient in lithotomy position with drape covering legs	4
	C. Advise patient with each step of the exam so that she knows what to expect	5
	D. Have all equipment within arm's reach	6
IV.	INSPECTION	
	A. Ask the patient to allow her knees to fall out to side	7
	B. Depress drape toward the abdomen so that you can see the patient's face	8
	C. Position light source to illuminate the genitalia	9
	D. External genitalia	
	1. Note Sexual Maturity Rating[6]	
	a. Stage 1—no pubic hair	10
	b. Stage 2—scant fine hair growth	11
	c. Stage 3—hair becomes darker and coarse	12
	d. Stage 4—adult hair without spread to inner thighs	13
	e. Stage 5—spread to inner thighs	14
	2. Identify structure	
	a. Mons pubis	15
	b. Vulva	16
	c. Labia majora	17
	d. Perineum	18
	e. Anus	19
	3. Identify abnormalities	
	a. Skin changes: lesions, rashes, atrophy	20
	b. Parasites	21
	4. Advise patient you are going to touch her and separate the labia majora	22
	a. Clitoris	23
	b. Inspect the urethral meatus	24
	c. Introitus	25
	d. Labia minor	26
	e. Identify: lesions, discharge	27
	5. Advise patient you will be touching the vaginal opening	28
	a. Place two fingers at the posterior introitus	29
	b. Have the patient bare down	30
	c. Examine for rectocele, urethrocele, glandular enlargement	31
V.	PALPATION	
	A. Milk urethra for discharge	32

FEMALE GENITALIA AND RECTUM FLOW

Flow #12

Performed

	B.	Palpate secretory glands for enlargement or tenderness		
		1.	Bartholin gland	33
		2.	Skene gland	34
	C.	Place one finger into the vagina and note position of the cervix		35
VI.	SPECULUM EXAMINATION			
	A.	Advise patient that you are now going to place a speculum into the vagina		36
	B.	Prepare speculum by testing function and warming with warm water		37
	C.	Place two fingers in the posterior introitus and press downward		38
	D.	Introduce speculum: blades closed, vertically oriented, and at a 45-degree downward angle and rotate to horizontal		39
	E.	Inspection		
		1.	Bring cervix into view and lock speculum in place	40
		2.	Note anatomy and abnormalities	
			a. Squamocolumnar junction, shape of os, color	41
			b. Lesions, discharge	42
		3.	Perform PAP smear at squamocolumnar junction and obtain endocervical sample	43
		4.	Unlock blades	44
			a. Remove speculum slowly while closing blades	45
			b. Inspect vaginal walls for lesions, discharge	46
VII.	BIMANUAL EXAMINATION			
	A.	Stand at end of bed		47
	B.	Advise that you will be inserting two fingers into the vagina		48
	C.	Lubricate fingers		49
	D.	Insert fingers with thumb retracted to avoid contact with the clitoris		50
	E.	Palpate cervix and assess for cervical motion tenderness		51
	F.	Assess height and position of the uterus with free hand depressing the abdomen		52
	G.	Palpate the adnexa for masses, tenderness		53
	H.	Perform rectovaginal exam		
		1.	Change gloves	54
		2.	Advise patient rectal examination will now be performed	55
		3.	Insert one lubricated finger into rectum and one finger intervaginally	56
		4.	Palpate the posterior vaginal wall	57
		5.	Remove vaginal finger, palpate the rectal wall in 360 degrees for masses	58

NOTES:

MALE GENITALIA AND RECTUM FLOW

Flow #13

Performed

I.	INTRODUCES SELF		1
II.	EXPLAINS that physical exam will now be performed.		2
III.	PATIENT EDUCATION		
	A.	Instruct on testicular self examination (TSE)	2
	B.	Advise rectal exams are recommended starting at age 50 and assess for prostatic and colorectal cancer.	3
	C.	Advise colonoscopy at 50 years of age or with family history of colorectal cancer, 10 years prior to the age of relative's diagnosis.	4
IV.	PREPARATION		
	A.	Explain that genital exam will now be performed.	5
	B.	Consider having an additional attendant in room.	6
	C.	Glove.	7
	D.	Have patient expose the genital area.	8
V.	GENITAL EXAMINATION		
	A.	Inspection	
		1. Have patient stand or lie in supine position.	9
		2. Have patient bear down and observe inguinal area for bulging.	10
		3. Note Sexual Maturity Rating[7]	
		a. Stage 1—no pubic hair	11
		b. Stage 2—scant fine hair growth	12
		c. Stage 3—hair becomes darker and coarse	13
		d. Stage 4—adult hair without spread to inner thighs	14
		e. Stage 5—spread to inner thighs	15
		4. Identify abnormalities	
		a. Skin changes: lesions, rashes	16
		b. Parasites	17
	B.	Inspection and palpation of the penis	
		1. Retract prepuce if present. Note lesions or exudate. Detract when completed.	18
		2. Inspect the urethral meatus. Note position and discharge.	19
		3. Inspect the penile shaft and glans. Note deformity or lesions.	20
		4. Palpate shaft for masses.	21
		5. Palpate urethra from proximal to distal and assess meatal discharge.	22
	C.	Inspection of scrotum—note lesions, masses.	23
		a. Note size and shape.	24
		b. Note nodules and tenderness.	25

MALE GENITALIA AND RECTUM FLOW

Flow #13

Performed

D.		Inspection and palpation of the testicles.	
	1.	Note which testicle descends further.	26
	2.	Palpate testes between thumb and pads of first two fingers.	27
	3.	Palpate epididymis noting masses and tenderness.	28
	4.	Palpate spermatic cord working proximally.	29
E.		Palpate for inguinal hernia	
	1.	Invaginate scrotum with index finger. Palpate external inguinal ring.	30
	2.	Use right finger for right side and left finger for left side.	31
	3.	Have patient turn head and cough. Assess for hernias.	32
VI.		RECTAL EXAMINATION	
	A.	Have patient bend over exam table, or lie in the lateral decubitus position.	33
	B.	Inspection of perineum and anus	
	1.	Note lesions, fissures, rashes, hemorrhoids.	34
	2.	Have patient bear down and observe anal orifice.	35
	C.	Palpation	
	1.	Apply lubrication to finger	36
	2.	Advise patient you will be touching the anus.	37
	3.	Place pad of finger on anus.	38
	4.	Have patient bear down and then relax.	39
	5.	Upon relaxation, insert finger into the anus with pad of finger anteriorly.	40
		a. Note sphincter tone	41
		b. Palpate prostate—note size, shape, consistency, nodules and tenderness.	42
		c. Rotate finger 360 degrees and palpate rectal wall for lesions.	43
	6.	Retract finger and perform occult blood test.	44
	7.	Clean anus with tissue.	45
VII.		CLINICAL SCENARIO	
	A.	Scrotal mass	
	1.	Auscultate for bowel sounds	46
	2.	Transilluminate	47
	B.	Hernia detected on scrotal invagination.	
	1.	Tap on tip of finger—may indicate indirect inguinal hernia	48
	2.	Tap on side of finger—may indicate direct inguinal hernia	49

NOTES:

References

1. Seidel, HM. *Mosby's Guide to Physical Examination*, 5th ed. St. Louis: Mosby; 2006: 439.

2. Swartz, MH. *Textbook of Physical Diagnosis: History and Examination*, 5th ed. Philadelphia, PA: Saunders; 2006: 671–680.

3. Swartz, MH. *Textbook of Physical Diagnosis: History and Examination*, 5th ed. Philadelphia, PA: Saunders; 2006: 680.

4. Swartz, MH. *Textbook of Physical Diagnosis: History and Examination*, 5th ed. Philadelphia, PA: Saunders; 2006: 689.

5. Bickley, LS. *Bates Guide to Physical Examination and History Taking*, 9th ed. Philadelphia, PA: Lippincott Williams & Wilkins; 2007: 779.

6. Bickley, LS. *Bates Guide to Physical Examination and History Taking*, 9th ed. Philadelphia, PA: Lippincott Williams & Wilkins; 2007: 783.

7. Bickley, LS. *Bates Guide to Physical Examination and History Taking*, 9th ed. Philadelphia, PA: Lippincott Williams & Wilkins; 2007: 781.

COMPREHENSIVE FLOWS:
BRINGING IT ALL
TOGETHER

5

This chapter pulls together the concepts you learned in Chapters 1 through 3 about history taking and Chapter 4, which covers the physical examination. Students who took excellent histories and performed detailed exam Flows may now find it quite difficult to bring the two together. The comprehensive Flows encourage the practitioner to identify the most important aspects of each system Flow. For example, in the patient with suspected hypertension, the vital signs would be completed followed by an ophthalmoscopic examination looking for evidence of hypertensive changes. There would be little else in the HEENT system that would merit examination in this problem specific case. You would not check this patient's hearing. With time, you will be able to perform a limited, problem specific examination, honing the skills of observation into a precise collection of physical findings related only to the presenting complaints.

The Comprehensive Flow is designed to be another partnered practical examination. Again, one student is the provider who performs the history and physical, while the other takes on the role of the patient. You may perform the first several cases without a time limit; however, after the first few cases, you should be able to progress to accomplishing your tasks within the time limits set forth below.

Each case starts with the provider receiving a face sheet that contains the patient's name, clinical setting, and chief complaint. It also provides the vital signs. This simulates office settings where triage is performed by other staff members. It is very important to review the vital signs and repeat them if needed. For example, if the face sheet shows a blood pressure of 140/85 mmHg in a person who is diabetic, it would be important to repeat the blood pressure as the goal for blood pressure in diabetics is less than 130/80 mmHg (**BQ**). You may be elated when a patient who has known hypertension with very poor control, returns and has a screening blood pressure that is normal. But your elation may soon be deflated as your repeat pressure shows 180/100. Performing the measurements yourself is always a good idea.

Once the provider has read the face sheet, the history taking begins. The provider will have 14 minutes to elicit a history and perform the problem-specific physical examination. These time limits are meant to reflect a typical outpatient visit. Within the later half of this period, the provider should share the differential diagnosis with the patient and advise them of the plan, asking if they have any questions, and finally thank the patient for the visit. At the end of the visit, the provider should write a SOAP note within a 9-minute limit.

A question arises about washing one's hands. Providers are the most likely source of disease transmission in the patient setting. When entering a room, courtesy often dictates shaking the person's hand. However, if you just left the prior room and did not wash your hands upon exiting—a mistake that should be avoided—and you then shake your new patient's hand, you have now spread whatever was on your hands from the patient you saw earlier to your current patient. She came in with acid reflux and left with pink eye. A good technique as you enter the room is to explain that you just have to wash your hands before shaking theirs, or because many institutions now have antibacterial cleaners outside of each room, enter the room rubbing the cleanser in. In either case, the patient will appreciate your efforts to keep him or her healthy.

Review of the Strategy

The history component stays essentially the same. If you get lost, fall back on the CODIERSM-MASSH mnemonic. The physical examination, however, must now be problem-specific. If, for example, the patient comes in with shortness of breath and you think it is likely that they have congestive heart failure, you would need to examine multiple systems but in a problem-focused approach. Having been given the vital signs, you would complete the general assessment, looking for position of comfort and respiratory distress. You would look for pallor, cyanosis, and clubbing in the integumentary system as well as the neck for JVD. The majority of your exam would concentrate on the cardiac and respiratory exams looking for heart murmurs, S3 and S4, and crackles. You would perform a hepatojugular reflex and look for peripheral edema.

It is obvious that you will not have time to examine each of these flows in their entirety, so you must pick and choose the most fruitful parts of each flow to incorporate into your problem-specific exam.

Finally, it is recognized that many more questions could be asked for each Flow as well as additional components of the exams being performed. The Flows are designed to provide answers to high yield inquiries and components of the exam. Again, prepare three possibilities for your differential diagnosis. Some cases may not have a distinct diagnosis but possibility of several.

To perform the Comparative Flow:

1. Pair into partners with one in the provider role and the other in the patient role.
2. The patient reads the Flow to become familiar with the problem and the answers.
3. The provider begins taking the history and performing problem-specific examination with a 14-minute time limit.
4. Educate the patient about the likely diagnosis and the plan for evaluation and treatment.
5. Switch partners and begin a new case with same time limits.
6. At the end of the second case, both students should write a SOAP note with a 9-minute time limit.

PATIENT NAME: EBNER WAY
Clinical Setting: Primary Care Office

Case Information: An 88 y/o male presents with back pain
Vital Signs
Blood pressure: 152/72
Respirations: 16 per minute
Pulse: 70 bpm
Temperature: 98.2°F
Weight: 166 lbs
Height: 5'9"
Pain: 4 or 5

PATIENT NAME: EBNER WAY
Clinical Setting: Primary Care Office

Subjective

Objective

Assessment

Plan

CC: A 88 y/o male presents with back pain

History   Performed

	1	Introduces self.	
	2	Explains role of provider.	
	3	Opening question: What brings you in today?	My back hurts.
Chronology/ Onset	4	**How** did you hurt it?	I slipped on the rug and fell on my butt.
	5	**When** did that happen?	Last night.
	6	Did this ever happen **before**?	No.
Description/ Duration	7	**Describe** the pain.	I don't know, it just hurts.
	8	**Where** is the pain?	Right in the middle, on my butt bone.
Intensity	9	Rate the **intensity** on a scale of 1 to 10?	A 4 or 5.
Exacerbation	10	What makes it **worse**?	Sitting on it.
Remission	11	What makes it **better**?	Nothing, that's why I'm here.
Symptoms	12	Any **swelling**?	I can't see back there.
associated	13	Any change to your **bowel or bladder** habits?	No. I'm as regular as Old Faithful.
	14	Any **incontinence**?	Nope.
	15	Any **numbness, weakness or tingling**?	Nope.
Medical Hx	16	Any **medical conditions**?	I've got high blood pressure and gout.
Medications	17	What **medications** are you on?	A water pill and gout pill.
Allergies	18	Do you have any **allergies**?	Nope.
Surgical Hx	19	Any previous **operations**?	No.

Physical Examination

	20	Informs patient that the physical exam is to begin.	
	21	Washes hands for 15 seconds.	
Vitals	22	Performs repeat vitals if appropriate.	Repeat bp 138/84.
General	23	Assess for **distress from pain**.	Patient standing, will not sit.
MS	24	Examines the spine.	

				Performed
	25	Inspection: **Errythema, ecchymosis, edema**	Ecchimosis at inferior sacrum.	
	26	Palpation: **Warmth, tenderness, edema**	Tenderness at midsacrum.	
	27	Osteopathic examination	Right on right sacral torsion.	
Neuro	28	Lower extremity **reflexes**	2/4 bilateral patellar and achilles	
	29	Lower extremity **strength**	5/5 hip and knee flexion/extension	
Assessment/	30	Give three things in the differential diagnosis including sacral torsion.		
Plan	31	Explained plan: pain control, manipulation, radiologic exam.		
	32	Perform appropriate manipulation.		
	33	Asks the patient if he has any questions.		
	34	Thanks the patient. Displayed professionalism and empathy.		

Case Review #1

This is an 88-year-old man presenting with back pain after slipping on a rug and falling the previous night. The history of trauma points you immediately toward a musculoskeletal etiology; however, do not discount other possibilities. One elderly gentleman presented to the ER with abdominal pain after a fall. He was sure that he had just pulled a muscle but a 6.5 cm abdominal aortic aneurysm was found.

The patient locates the pain in the sacral area. Symptoms associated should include changes in bowel or bladder habits, a new onset of incontinence or numbness, tingling or weakness, which should lead you to expand your differential diagnosis and may require an immediate surgical consult.

When asked what makes his pain better, the patient states, "Nothing." The questioning should be expanded to define what exactly he has tried for it.

The patient has a history of HTN. The initial blood pressure measurement was 152/72. Since the systolic reading was high, a repeat blood pressure should be performed. The repeat BP of 138/84 is at the goal of less than 140/90 based on his past medical history. Had he had a diagnosis of diabetes or renal insufficiency, his blood pressure goal would be at < 130/80. These values are Board questions (**BQ**).

The patient will not sit because of the pain, but his lower extremity reflexes and strength are intact on physical exam. If a patient in unable or unwilling to perform part of an examination, the provider must improvise to get the best possible examination. If you ask this patient if he can sit for 30 seconds, you should be able to check his reflexes. If he still claims he cannot sit, ask the patient how he got to the office. He likely sat in some fashion; replicate it.

The evaluation and treatment should include imaging and pain management. The patient should be advised to take an anti-inflammatory for pain control. The risks and side effects of the medication should be discussed and properly documented in the chart.

PATIENT NAME: ROSIE OSE
Clinical Setting: Primary Care Office

A 21 y/o female complaining of a cold
Vital Signs
Blood pressure: 110/60
Respirations: 16 per minute
Pulse: 72 bpm
Temperature: 100.1°F
Weight: 128 lbs
Height: 5'9"
Pain: 0 out of 10

PATIENT NAME: ROSIE OSE
Clinical Setting: Primary Care Office

Subjective

Objective

Assessment

Plan

CC: A 21 y/o female presents to the family practice office c/o "a cold"

History			Performed
	1	Introduces self.	
	2	Explains role of provider.	
	3	Opening question: What brings you in today?	I've got a cold.
Chronology/ Onset	4	When did it **start**?	About 3 days ago.
	5	Was the onset **sudden** or **gradual**?	I guess gradual.
	6	Did you ever have this **before**?	I had the same thing last year.
Description	7	**Describe** the "cold."	I have a clear runny nose and sore throat.
Exacerbations	8	Anything make it **worse**?	It hurts more when I swallow.
Remittance	9	Anything make it **better**?	Some cold tablets I took helped.
Symptoms associated	10	Do you have any **shortness of breath**?	I just can't breathe through my nose.
	11	**Fever or chills**?	Both.
	12	**Headache** or sinus congestion/pressure?	Yes, right above my eyes.
	13	Do you have any **visual changes**?	No.
	14	Any **ear pain**?	No, they just feel full.
	15	Do you have a **cough**?	No.
Medical Hx	16	Do you have any other **medical conditions**?	No, I'm pretty healthy.
Medications	17	What **medications** are you on?	None.
Allergies	18	Do you have any **allergies**?	I'm allergic to amoxicillin.
	19	What happens when you take that?	I vomit.
Social Hx	20	Do you **smoke**?	No.
Menstrual Hx	21	When was the **FDLNMP**?	It started yesterday.
Surg/Hosp Hx	22	Have you had any **surgeries** or **hospitalizations**?	No.

Physical Exam

	23	Informs patient that the physical exam is to begin.	
	24	Washes hands for 15 seconds.	
Vitals	25	Appropriately performed—if repeated measurements needed.	
General	26	General assessment	Alert, no respiratory distress.
Skin	27	Rash	None.
Head/Sinuses	28	Inspection, palpation	Normocephalic, atraumatic. Sinuses nontender.

			Performed
Eyes	29	Inspection	Conjunctive pink, sclera w/o injection
Nose	30	Inspection	Mucosal edema and clear exudate
Ears	31	Inspection	TMs gray bilaterally, good light reflex
Mouth/Throat	32	Inspection	Pharyngeal erythema w/o exudate
Neck/Lymph	33	Inspection, palpation	Supple without masses, lymphadenopathy, or stiffness.
Lungs	34	Auscultation	Clear without wheezes, crackles
Cardiac	35	Auscultation: aortic, pulmonic, tricuspid, and mitral	Regular without murmur
Abdomen	36	Palpation	No splenomegaly.
Assessment/	37	Give three things in the differential diagnosis including URI.	
Plan	38	Explained likely etiology: Viral infection.	
	39	Explained plan: supportive therapy, throat culture, increase fluids, rest.	
	40	Asks the patient and family if they have any questions or suggestions.	
	41	Thanks the patient. Displayed professionalism and empathy.	

Case Review #2

This is a 21-year-old healthy female presenting to the office with a "cold." Upon seeing the chief complaint on the triage sheet, you develop a differential diagnosis before entering the room. The differential diagnosis includes an upper respiratory tract infection, pharyngitis, or otitis media and sinusitis, either bacterial or viral.

Early in the interview, you should define what a "cold" means to the patient. This essentially allows you to expand on the symptoms associated. Medical providers often use the term interchangeably with an upper respiratory tract infection (URI).

The patient states that her symptoms started 3 days ago and that she had a similar episode a year ago. Despite the benign early appearance, finding an increase frequency of colds could alert the provider to an immunodeficiency.

As with all female patients, it is important to note when the patient's FDLNMP and her allergies in the event that the patient needs antibiotics for a bacterial infection.

On physical exam, the patient is alert and respirations are not labored. The nasal mucosa is edematous and clear exudate is present. The tympanic membranes are not inflamed. The pharynx is erythematous and without exudate. The physical findings along with the short duration of the symptoms point to the diagnosis of a viral URI.

The plan may include a throat culture to rule out a bacterial pharyngitis. The patient should be advised that if the throat culture is positive, she will be placed on an antibiotic at that time. She should be encouraged to increase her fluid intake and rest. Decongestants and anti-inflammatory medications can be used for symptomatic relief.

Most upper respiratory infections are viral but it is difficult to differentiate between viral and bacterial infections. Signs and symptoms of bacterial and viral URIs are often indistinguishable. Clinical judgment must be relied upon to determine whether a URI is viral or bacterial.

PATIENT NAME: PAINE SHRODER
Clinical Setting: Primary Care Office

A 48 y/o male with left shoulder pain
Vital Signs
Blood pressure: 126/70
Respirations: 16 per minute
Pulse: 68 bpm
Temperature: 98.2°F
Weight: 188 lbs
Height: 6'1"
Pain: 6 to 7

PATIENT NAME: PAINE SHRODER
Clinical Setting: Primary Care Office

Subjective

Objective

Assessment

Plan

CC: A 48 y/o male presents with left shoulder pain

History   Performed

	1 Introduces self.	
	2 Explains the role of the provider.	
	3 Opening question: What brings you in today?	My left shoulder hurts.
Chronology/	4 How did you hurt it?	I was probably just over using it.
Onset	5 When did you first notice it?	For a couple of weeks.
	6 Did this ever happen before?	No.
Description/	7 Describe the pain.	It's just like a bad toothache.
Duration	8 Where is the pain?	In my whole shoulder.
Intensity	9 Intensity on a scale of 1 to 10?	A 6 or 7.
Exacerbation	10 What makes it worse?	Trying to lift my arm over my head.
Remission	11 What makes it better?	Icy-Hot helped a bit.
Symptoms	12 Any swelling?	No.
associated	13 Is the range of motion limited?	Yes, it hurts to move it.
	14 Any numbness, weakness or tingling?	No.
	15 Any chest pain, nausea, vomiting, SOB?	No.
Medical Hx	16 Any medical conditions (HTN, dyslipidemia)?	No.
Medications	17 What medications are you on?	None.
Allergies	18 Do you have any allergies?	Just to bee stings.
Social Hx	19 How did you overuse it/what is your job?	I'm a roofer.
	20 Do you smoke?	No.
Surgical Hx	21 Any previous operations?	No.
Family Hx	22 Heart attack or stroke in their 50s or younger?	No.

Physical Examination

	23 Informs patient that the physical exam is to begin.	
	24 Washes hands for 15 seconds.	

			Performed
Vitals	25	Performs repeat vitals if appropriate.	
General	26	Assess for **distress from pain**.	No distress.
MS	27	Performs complete shoulder examination **bilaterally**.	
	28	Inspection: **Errythema, ecchymosis, edema**	None
	29	Palpation: **Warmth, tenderness, edema**	Tenderness at superspinatus
	30	Range of Motion: **Active/passive flexion/extension**	ROM limited by pain
	31	Special tests: **Drop arm test**	Negative
Heart	32	Inspection	No heave
	33	Palpation	PMI 5th ICS-MCL
	34	Auscultation	No murmur, rub, or gallop
Lungs	35	Auscultation	Clear to auscultation
Assessment/	36	Give three things in the differential diagnosis including strain.	
Plan	37	Explained plan: pain control, physical therapy, local therapy.	
	38	Perform appropriate manipulation including Spencer techniques.	
	39	Asks the patient if he has any questions.	
	40	Thanks the patient. Displayed professionalism and empathy.	

Case Review #3

This is a 48-year-old roofer who presents with left shoulder pain. The patient's pain is exacerbated when he lifts his arm over his head. He believes that he may just have been overusing the arm. Although listening to your patents is important, other more serious causes of the shoulder pain must be considered. Your differential diagnosis initially should include musculoskeletal etiology and myocardial infarction.

The patient has had pain for the past couple weeks and denies chest pain, nausea, and SOB. The patient does not smoke or have a history of HTN or dyslipidemia, which makes a cardiac cause less likely. He is a roofer and may indeed have an overuse syndrome.

On physical exam, there is tenderness at the supraspinatus and range of motion (ROM) is limited by pain. The drop arm test is negative, which makes the diagnosis of rotator cuff tear less likely. With pain on movement and palpation, a cardiac etiology is very unlikely.

The patient should be treated conservatively with therapy localized to the shoulder, such as heat or topical analgesic and anti-inflammatory medications. Manipulation should include Spencer techniques. The patient should initate and participate in range of motion exercises at home or be referred to physical therapy.

PATIENT NAME: OCTAVE HIGHER
Clinical Setting: ER

A 14 y/o male presents to the ER with pain

Vital Signs

Blood pressure: 140/86

Respirations: 32 per minute

Pulse: 120 bpm

Temperature: 99.0°F

Weight: 142 lbs

Height: 6'

Pain: 10 out of 10

PATIENT NAME: OCTAVE HIGHER
Clinical Setting: ER

Subjective

Objective

Assessment

Plan

A 14 y/o male presents to the ER with pain

History

			Performed
	1	Introduces self.	
	2	Explains the role of the provider.	
	3	Opening question: What brings you in today?	I've got a terrible pain in my groin.
Chronology/	4	When did it **start**?	About a half hour ago.
Onset	5	Did you ever have this **before**?	Never.
	6	Did it come on **suddenly or gradually**?	Suddenly.
	7	What were you **doing** at the time?	I was running with a football.
	8	Was there any **trauma**?	No, I was just running.
	9	Has it **changed**?	It's getting worse and worse.
Description	10	**Describe the pain.**	It's just horrible, like a giant squeeze.
	11	**Where** is the pain?	Points to the *scrotum*.
Intensity	12	How severe is it, on a scale from **1 to 10**?	It's a 15.
Exacerbations	13	What makes it **worse**?	If you touch it at all or I move.
Remittance	14	What makes it **better**?	No. Please help me.
Symptoms	15	Any **nausea or vomiting**?	I feel like I want to vomit.
associated	16	**Fever or chills**?	I don't think so.
	17	**Penile discharge**?	No.
Medical Hx	18	Do you have any other **medical conditions**?	No.
Medications	19	Are you on any **medications**?	No.
Allergies	20	Do you have any **allergies**?	No.
Social Hx	21	Are you **sexually active**?	No.
Surgical Hx	22	Any prior **surgeries**?	I had a hydrocele fixed when I was four.
Hospitalizations	23	Any prior **hospitalizations**?	Just for my surgery.

Physical Exam

	24	Informs patient that the physical exam is to begin.	
	25	Washes hands for 15 seconds.	

			Performed
Vitals	26	Performs repeat vitals if appropriate.	Repeat BP 146/90, R 32, P 120
General	27	General assessment	Alert, unable to find position of comfort.
Respiratory	28	Auscultation: symmetrically.	Clear to auscultation
Cardiac	29	Auscultation: aortic, pulmonic, tricuspid, and mitral	RRR w/o murmur, rub, or gallop
Abdominal	30	Inspection	Scaphoid
	31	Auscultation	Normoactive bowel sounds
	32	Palpation	Nontender, without masses
Genital	33	Inspection	Scrotum enlarged, erythematous, and edematous.
	34	Palpation	Exquisitely tender left testicle lying transversely and high in the scrotum.
Assessment	35	Explained differential diagnosis including **testicular torsion**.	
Plan	36	Explained pathophysiology: **twisting of testes** and cord with acute ischemia.	
	37	Explained plan: ultrasound, manual reduction, surgical consult.	
	38	Asks the patient if he has any questions or suggestions.	
	39	Thanks the patient. Displayed professionalism and empathy throughout the interview.	

Case Review #4

This is a 14-year-old presenting with a sudden onset of scrotal pain that began while he was running with a football. The patient denies actual trauma such as being tackled. The initial differential diagnosis could include muscle strain, testicular torsion, orchitis, epididymitis, and incarcerated hernia.

The history shows a sudden onset of extreme pain in the scrotum made worse with movement or palpation. He is not sexually active and denies penile discharge, which makes an infectious process less likely. He does have a past surgical history for hydrocele repair, which leads to consideration of possible pelvic diaphragm weakness or scar tissue.

On exam, the testicle is extremely tender and is lying transverse and high in the scrotum, which is a classical finding for testicular torsion (**BQ**). If the testicle was in a normal position, epididymitis would have been of higher consideration.

The twisting of the testes and cord causes acute ischemia and is a surgical emergency. An ultrasound should be performed and urologist should be consulted immediately in order to attempt to save the testicle. Surgical detorsion may be required.

PATIENT NAME: JIM HUBERT
Clinical Setting: Family Practice Outpatient Office

A 48 y/o male presents with foot pain
Vital Signs
Blood pressure: 158/92
Respirations: 12 per minute
Pulse: 92 bpm
Temperature: 99.0°F
Weight: 210 lbs
Height: 6'1"
Pain: 8 out of 10

PATIENT NAME: JIM HUBERT
Clinical Setting: Family Practice Outpatient Office

Subjective

Objective

Assessment

Plan

CC: A 48 y/o male presents with foot pain

History			Performed
	1	Introduces self.	
	2	Explains the role of the provider.	
	3	Opening question: What brings you in today?	My foot is killing me.
Chronology/ Onset	4	**When** did it start?	It woke me up out of dead sleep last night.
	5	Did you ever have this pain **before**?	Once, last year, but it only lasted a day.
	6	Was there any **trauma**?	Not that I can think of.
Description/	7	**Describe** the pain.	It feels like it is on fire.
Duration	8	**Where** is the pain?	It's all in my right big toe.
Intensity	9	**Any other areas/radiation**?	No.
Exacerbation	10	Intensity on a scale of 1 to 10?	I'd say it's at least an 8.
Remission	11	What makes it **worse**?	Touching it. Even the sheet hurts it.
Symptoms associated	12	What makes it **better**?	Nothing. I tried some acetaminophen.
	13	Any **swelling**?	Yes, a little.
	14	Any **redness**?	Yes, a lot.
	15	Any **increased heat**?	Yes, it's hot.
	16	Any **fever or chills**?	Maybe a little.
Medical Hx	17	Do you have any other **medical conditions**?	I have high blood pressure.
Medications	18	What **medications** are you on?	I'm on a water pill.
Allergies	19	Do you have any **allergies**?	No.
Surgical Hx	20	Any previous **operations**?	I just had my gallbladder out last week.
Social Hx	21	Do you **smoke**?	No.
	22	Do you drink **alcohol**?	Yes.
	23	How much a day?	Oh, 4 or 5 beers.

Physical Examination

	24	Informs patient that the physical exam is to begin.
	25	Washes hands for 15 seconds.

			Performed
Vitals	26	Correctly performs repeat vitals if appropriate.	
General	27	Assess for **distress from pain**.	No grimace while sitting.
Skin	28	Inspection: Bilateral lower extremity **Erythema, ecchymosis, edema, lesions.**	Right foot erythema concentrated around 1st MTP joint to inferior medial malleolus. +1 foot edema.
	29	Palpation: Assess for **warmth w/ back of hands**	Increase warmth at 1st MTP.
Respiratory	30	Auscultation	Clear without wheezes or crackles.
Cardiac	31	Auscultation	Regular w/o murmur, rub, or gallop.
Extremity	32	Inspection **Boney deformity/ arthritic changes.**	None.
	33	Palpation **Tenderness**	Exquisitely tender to light palpation
Vascular/Peripheral	34	Palpation **Bilateral peripheral pulses.**	Dorsalis pedis and post tibialis 2/4
	35	**Capillary refill.**	<1 second
Assessment/	36	Give three things in the differential diagnosis including gout.	
Plan	37	Explained likely pathophysiology: excessive uric acid production.	
	38	Explained plan: imaging, labs with uric acid level, pharmacological rxn (pain and gout).	
	39	Provides education: Diet modification, decrease alcohol, change to nondiuretic bp rxn.	
	40	Thanks the patient and asks if there are questions. Displayed professionalism.	

Case Review #5

The patient presents complaining of foot pain, but specifically asking where the pain is shows that the pain is localized in the right great toe. Immediately, gout should become higher in the differential diagnosis. There is a small hint of a prior occurrence, which appears to have been self-limited.

The patient has several risk factors for gout: being on a diuretic for his blood pressure, which may well be hydrocholothiazide, he has had a recent operation, and he drinks alcohol. On examination, we find errythema and swelling surrounding the first metatarsalphalangeal joint.

The diagnosis of gout can be pursued by ordering a uric acid level. Imaging may also be done and pain relief is the patient's primary concern.

PATIENT NAME: SHERRY CALLAWAY
Clinical Setting: Outpatient Primary Care Office

A 49 y/o female presents to the office with a rash
Vital Signs
Blood pressure: 118/58
Respirations: 12 per minute
Pulse: 72 bpm
Temperature: 98.8°F
Weight: 132 lbs
Height: 5'4"
Pain: 0 out of 10

PATIENT NAME: SHERRY CALLAWAY
Clinical Setting: Outpatient Primary Care Office

Subjective

Objective

Assessment

Plan

CC: A 49 y/o female presents to the office with a rash

History

			Performed
	1	Introduces self.	
	2	Explains the role of the provider.	
	3	Opening question: What brings you in today?	I have a rash.
Chronology/	4	When did it **start**?	About a week ago.
Onset	5	Did you ever have this **before**?	No.
Description	6	**Where** did the rash **start**?	It started on my wrist.
	7	Did it **spread** anywhere else?	It's all over, even my breasts.
	8	What does it **look like**?	It's all red and bumpy.
Exacerbations	9	Anything make it **worse**?	It's really bad at night.
Remittance	10	Anything make it **better**?	I tried an oatmeal bath but it didn't help.
Symptoms	11	Does it **itch**?	It itches like crazy.
associated	12	**Fever or chills**?	No.
	13	Recent **colds**?	No.
Medical Hx	14	Do you have any other **medical conditions**?	I'm starting to get some arthritis.
Medications	15	What **medications** are you on?	Just acetaminophen.
	16	Any **new medications**?	No.
Allergies	17	Do you have any **allergies**?	Aspirin upsets my stomach.
Social Hx	18	Any **contacts** with the same rash?	I think a couple of the patients have it.
	19	What patients?	I just started working at a nursing home.
	20	When was the FDLNMP?	I had a hysterectomy.
	21	Do you **smoke**?	Yes.
	22	**How much a day**?	About half a pack.
	23	Do you drink **alcohol** or use any **drugs**?	I'm too old for that.

Physical Exam

	24	Informs patient that the physical exam is to begin.	
	25	Washes hands for 15 seconds and puts gloves on.	
Vitals	26	Performs repeat vitals if appropriate.	
General	27	General assessment	Alert, no apparent distress
Integumentary	28	Inspection	Erythematous papules and excoriations

			Performed
	29	Includes web spaces of fingers	Burrows
	30	Includes areola with female assistant	1 mm vesicles and papules
HEENT	31	Inspection	TMs gray, throat w/o erythema nose w/o exudate
Lymph	32	Palpation	No cervical/axillary lymphadenopathy
Respiratory	33	Auscultation	Clear to auscultation
Cardiac	34	Auscultation	Regular rhythm w/o murmur, rub, or gallop
Assessment/	35	Explained differential diagnosis including scabies.	
Plan	36	Explained likely etiology: mite contacted at nursing home.	
	37	Explained plan: laundering all clothing and linen, topical lotion, antihistamine.	
	38	Educate nursing home staff of need to treat all contacts.	
	39	Asks the patient if she has any questions or suggestions.	
	40	Thanks the patient. Displayed professionalism and empathy throughout the interview.	

Case Review #6

This patient presents with a rash that started 1 week prior. It is important to note which area of the body the rash started on and where it traveled to. This aids in the differential diagnosis as certain disease processes follow particular patterns. For instance, the rash associated with Rocky Mountain Spotted Fever begins on the wrists and ankles, and then spreads to the trunk, palms, and sole. This is a (**BQ**).

Noting precise location is also important. Patients with neurodermatitis lack lesions where they cannot reach to excoriate themselves.

A contact history is crucial, not only to discern etiology of the rash but, if infectious, to contain it where it resides. This patient admits to starting a new job where some of the nursing home residents have a similar rash. Other contact questions should ask about new detergents, chemicals, or environmental exposures.

The physical exam should include a thorough examination of all skin areas including the scalp, ears, buccal mucosa, skin folds, trunk, and extremities. Lymphadenopathy can also aid in diagnosis. For example, a scalp rash with occipital nodes in pediatric patients alerts the provider to tinea capitis.

The key finding in this patient is burrows found in the web spaces of the hands. This is a (**BQ**).

Patient education must include notification of the suspected infestation to the nursing home so that the residents can be appropriately treated.

PATIENT NAME: NNEKA STRAIN
Clinical Setting: Family Practice Outpatient Office

A 49 y/o female presents with neck pain

Vital Signs

Blood pressure: 158/88

Respirations: 14 per minute

Pulse: 78 bpm

Temperature: 98.4°F

Weight: 156 lbs

Height: 5'3"

Pain: 7 out of 10

PATIENT NAME: NNEKA STRAIN
Clinical Setting: Family Practice Outpatient Office

Subjective

Objective

Assessment

Plan

CC: A 49 y/o female presents with neck pain

History

			Performed
	1	Introduces self.	
	2	Explains the role of the provider.	
	3	Opening question: What brings you in today?	My neck hurts.
Chronology/	4	**When** did it happen?	I just woke up like this today.
Onset	5	Have you ever had this **before**?	Yes, it acts up now and then.
	6	Any **activities** that could have hurt your neck?	Not that I know of.
Description/	7	**Describe** the pain.	It's just tight, and achy.
Duration	8	**Where** is the pain?	Right here (*grabs R superior trapezius*).
Intensity	9	**Intensity** on a scale of 1 to 10?	I'd say it's a 7.
Exacerbation	10	What makes it **worse**?	Moving my head too fast.
Remission	11	What makes it **better**?	If I massage it.
Symptoms	12	Any **trauma**?	I just must have slept on it wrong.
associated	13	Any **swelling, redness, or bruising**?	No.
	14	Is the **range of motion** limited?	Yes, I can't turn my head to the left.
	15	**Numbness or weakness** of the arms?	No.
	16	**Fever, chills, photophobia**?	No.
Medical Hx	17	Do you have any other **medical conditions**?	I had fibroids.
	18	When was the **FDLNMP**?	When they took my uterus out.
Medications	19	What **medications** are you on?	I just take a vitamin.
Allergies	20	Do you have any **allergies**?	No.
Surgical Hx	21	Any other previous **operations**?	Just my gallbladder when I was 38.

Physical Examination

	22	Informs patient that the physical exam is to begin.	
	23	Washes hands for 15 seconds.	
Vitals	24	Correctly repeats vitals if appropriate.	BP 156/86
General	25	Assess for **distress from pain**.	No distress
Head	26	Examines head	Normocephalic, atraumatic
Eyes	27	Funduscopic examination	No papilledema
Neck	28	Inspection	Symmetrical, trachea midline no masses, erythema, edema.

			Performed
	29	Palpation: musculoskeletal	Increased warmth, bogginess tenderness, at C5 transverse C5 Rotated Right, Side bent R
	30	Lymphatic	No lymphadenopathy
	31	Range of Motion	ROM limited by pain upon rotation or side bending to the left.
	32	Special tests: Kernig or Brudzinski test	Negative
Assessment/	33	Give three things in the differential diagnosis including cervical dysfunction/strain.	
Plan	34	Explained plan: NSAID, manipulation, exercises, return in 2 weeks for repeat blood pressure check.	
	35	Perform appropriate manipulation.	
	36	Asks the patient if she has any questions.	
	37	Thanks the patient. Displayed professionalism and empathy throughout the interview.	

Case Review #7

This is a 49-year-old female who woke up this morning with neck pain. Despite the obvious lack of immediately preceding trauma at the onset of pain, the provider should further question if there were any recent activities that may have caused the pain.

In a patient who presents with neck pain, it is important to rule out an infectious process such as meningitis. The patient denies fever, chills, and photophobia, which makes an infectious process less likely. Before meningitis is removed from your differential, you will need to carefully examine the neck during the physical exam.

The patient denies trauma, numbness, and weakness of the arms, which makes neurological involvement less likely.

On examination, the patient is afebrile and the Kernig and Brudzinski signs are negative. There is increased warmth, bogginess, and tenderness at the C5 transverse process and C5 is rotated to the right. These findings help to further rule out an infectious process and points to cervical somatic dysfunction or strain.

The patient's blood pressure is 158/88 and 156/86. The patient will need to be brought back to the office in 2 weeks for a second blood pressure check. The patient should be educated that HTN cannot be diagnosed with an isolated reading. The patient's blood pressure may be high as a result of her neck pain.

Manipulation should be explained to the patient and after obtaining a verbal consent performed on the patient. The patient should be advised to take an NSAID for pain control. The patient should be advised of the possible side effects of the medication and proper documentation of this discussion should be included in the patient's chart.

PATIENT NAME: EILEEN A. LITTLE
Clinical Setting: ER

An 82 y/o female is brought to the ER by ambulance
Vital Signs
Blood pressure: 186/112
Respirations: 12 per minute
Pulse: 84 bpm
Temperature: 98.4°F
Weight: 136 lbs
Height: 5'7"
Pain: 0 out of 10

PATIENT NAME: EILEEN A. LITTLE
Clinical Setting: ER

Subjective

Objective

Assessment

Plan

CC: 82 y/o female is brought to the ER by ambulance

History

			Performed
	1	Introduces self.	
	2	Explains the role of the provider.	
	3	Opening question: What brings you in today?	I feel weak.
Chronology/ Onset	4	When did it **start**?	About an hour ago.
	5	Was the onset **sudden** or **gradual**?	It happened all of a sudden.
	6	Did you ever have this **before**?	No.
Description	7	**Describe** the weakness.	It's my whole right side.
Symptoms associated	8	**Slurred speech, facial droop**?	No.
	9	**Numbness/tingling** on one side of your body?	My whole right side is numb, too.
	10	**Visual changes**?	I don't think so.
	11	**Headache**?	Not really.
	12	**Palpitations or chest pain**?	No.
	13	**Signs of breathing (SOB)**?	No.
	14	Have you had any **falls** recently?	No.
Medical Hx	15	Do you have any other **medical conditions**?	I have high blood pressure.
Medications	16	What **medications** are you on?	I'm supposed to be on something.
	17	Are you **taking your medications**?	Not all the time.
Allergies	18	Do you have any **allergies**?	No.
Social Hx	19	Do you **smoke**?	No.
	20	Do you drink **alcohol**?	No.
Surgical/Hosp Hx	21	Have you had any **surgeries** or **hospitalizations**?	No.

Physical Exam

	22	Informs patient that the physical exam is to begin.	
	23	Washes hands for 15 seconds.	
Vitals	24	Performs repeat vitals if appropriate.	Repeat BP 190/110
	25	Pulse for rate and rhythm	RR at 84 bpm
General	26	General assessment	Alert, no apparent distress
Neurologic	27	**Cranial nerves**: performs II-XII assessment	PERRLA, EOMI
			No facial droop, ptosis
			Uvula midline, rises midline
			Tongue midline when stuck out
			Shrugs shoulders equally
	28	**Muscle strength**: Bilateral upper extremities	Weaker right arm with drift

		Performed
	29 Bilateral lower extremities	Weaker right leg
	30 **Sensation**: Sharp and dull bilateral upper extremities	Diminished right arm
	31 Sharp and dull bilateral lower extremities	Diminished right leg
	32 **Reflexes**: bilateral upper and lower extremities	Decreased reflexes R arm and leg
	33 **Babinski**	Up going right, Down going left
Neck	34 Auscultation for bruits	Left carotid bruit
Cardiac	35 **Auscultation**: aortic, pulmonic, tricuspid, and mitral	2/6 systolic murmur aortic area
Respiratory	36 **Auscultation**: symmetrical approach	Clear to auscultation
Assessment/	37 Explained differential diagnosis including stroke	
Plan	38 Explained pathophysiology: Improper blood flow to the brain	
	39 Explained likely etiology: Carotid stenosis	
	40 Explained plan: Imaging (CT scan of the head), blood work, admission to the hospital	
	41 Asks the patient and family if they have any questions.	
	42 Thanks the patient. Displayed professionalism and empathy.	

Case Review #8

This is a 62-year-old female with a history of hypertension, brought to the ER for right-sided weakness. It is very important to develop the time frame, especially the onset of the patient's symptoms as the treatment plan is dependent on this information.

She has a sudden onset of unilateral weakness with paresthesias. This is a fairly classical presentation for stroke. The two most common causes of stroke are atrial fibrillation; hence, the patient should be asked about irregular or rapid heart beats, and carotid stenosis.

The patient has a risk factor of hypertension and admits noncompliance with her medications. Specifically, the patient should be asked if she takes an aspirin daily. Some people do not consider a baby aspirin a medication. She does not smoke.

The patient must be asked about recent surgeries as these may be a contraindication to fibrinolytic therapy.

On physical exam, a repeat BP is 190/110. A left carotid bruit is noted along with right-sided weakness of the upper and lower extremities. The focus should be on the neurologic examination. Reflexes are decreased in the upper and lower extremity with an up-going Babinski on the right. These findings indicate that the patient has had a stroke.

After explaining the diagnosis to the patient, the patient should be admitted to the hospital and a CT scan of the brain should be performed as soon as possible to determine if the stroke was caused by a bleed or by ischemia. After a bleed has been ruled out, the patient should be assessed for fibrinolytic therapy which should be given within 3 hours of the onset, again, stressing the importance of defining exactly when the symptoms started.

PATIENT NAME: SITTEN ONZACHEST
Clinical Setting: ER

A 59 y/o African American male presents to the ER with chest pain
Vital Signs
Blood pressure: 160/100
Respirations: 24 per minute
Pulse: 72 bpm
Temperature: 96.8°F
Weight: 230 lbs
Height: 5'11"
Pain: 8 out of 10

PATIENT NAME: SITTEN ONZACHEST
Clinical Setting: ER

Subjective

Objective

Assessment

Plan

CC: A 59 y/o African American male presents to the ER with chest pain

History			Performed
	1	Introduces self.	
	2	Explains the role of the provider.	
	3	Opening question: What brings you in today?	I have chest pain.
Chronology/ Onset	4	When did it **start**?	Two hours ago.
	5	What were you **doing when it started**?	Mowing the grass.
	6	Did you ever have this **before**?	Yes.
	7	When?	I seem to get it every time I mow.
	8	Was the onset **sudden** or **gradual**?	More gradual.
Description/	9	Is it **continuous** or does it **come and go**?	Continuous.
Duration	10	**Describe** the pain.	Like a crushing pain.
	11	**Where** is the pain?	*Points to left sternal border.*
	12	Does it **radiate** anywhere?	Up into my neck and left arm.
Intensity	13	Rate the **intensity** on a scale of 1 to 10?	An 8.
Exacerbation	14	What makes it **worse**?	Exerting myself.
Remission	15	What makes it **better**?	Resting.
Symptoms associated	16	Was there any sweating associated with it?	Yes.
	17	Do you have any **nausea or vomiting**?	No.
	18	**Shortness of breath**?	Maybe a little.
	19	**Dyspepsia**?	Maybe a little.
	20	**Cough**?	No.
Medical Hx	21	**Medical conditions** (HTN, hyperlipidemia, DM)?	Only high blood pressure.
Medications	22	What **medications** are you on?	Hydrochlorothiazide.
Allergies	23	Do you have any **allergies**?	No.
Social Hx	24	Do you **smoke**?	Yes.
	25	**How much** do you smoke a day?	Two packs a day.
	26	**How long** have you been smoking?	Ten years.
	27	Do you drink **alcohol**?	No.
	28	Do you use any **drugs**?	Just my prescription.
Family Hx	29	**Family with early heart attack or stroke**?	My Dad had a heart attack at 40.

Performed

Physical Examination

	30	Informs patient that the physical exam is to begin.	
	31	Washes hands for 15 seconds.	
Vitals	32	Correctly performs vital signs.	BP 160/96, P-100 reg, R-24
General	33	Assess for **distress**	No respiratory distress
Neck	34	Assess for **JVD**	No JVD
Cardiac	35	Inspection: **precordial heave**	No heave
	36	Palpation: Locate the PMI	Anterior axillary line 5th ICS
	37	Auscultation: **four areas** (aortic, pulmonic, tricuspid, and mitral)	
	38	With diaphragm and bell	
	39	Identify S1 and S2	Normal S1 and S2
	40	Identify murmurs, S3 and S4	No murmurs, S3 or S4
Respiratory	41	Inspection: **Labored, cyanosis, accessory muscle use**?	No respiratory distress
	42	Palpation: Reproducibility of **pain with palpation**	No tenderness
	43	Auscultation: **Instruct patient to breathe deeply through the mouth**	
	44	Through complete inspiration and expiration	Clear to auscultation
	45	Identify rhonchi, wheezes, crackles	
Abdomen	46	Inspection: **Pulsations**	No pulsations
	47	Palpation: pulsitile masses	No masses
Extremities	48	Inspection: edema	No edema
Assessment	49	Give three things in the differential diagnosis including myocardial infarction.	
Plan	50	Explained plan: stat chest X-ray, ECG, cardiac profile, aspirin, beta-blocker.	
	51	Explained pathophysiology: abnormality in perfusion of the heart.	
	52	Asks the patient if he has any questions.	
	53	Thanks the patient. Displayed professionalism and empathy throughout the interview.	

Case Review #9

This is a 59-year-old African-American male presenting to the ER with chest pain, which began while he was mowing the lawn. The patient describes the pain as occurring every time he mows. This leads you to think of angina and coronary artery disease. It is worse upon exertion and improves with rest, which is typical of angina. The description is of crushing chest pain suggesting visceral pain.

It is important to determine the patient's risk for coronary artery disease through historical questions. The patient is on medications for high blood pressure, smokes, and has a family history of heart disease. Additionally the patient is male.

The patient's vital signs should be repeated to ensure accuracy. The BP is high, he is tachypneic, and his pulse is 100 beats per minute showing some level of stress.

On physical exam the patient's level of discomfort should be noted. The patient should be assessed for signs of heart failure such as JVD, an S3, crackles in the lungs and edema, and an enlarged heart by a displaced point of maximal impulse (PMI).

This patient's historical and physical findings point to pain of a cardiac origin. He should be treated as having a myocardial infarction until proven otherwise. The patient should be given aspirin and started on a beta-blocker. He should have a stat chest X-ray, ECG, and a cardiac profile. He may need emergent assessment the coronary vasculature by catheterization.

NOTES:

PATIENT NAME: IZA ICHEN
Clinical Setting: Outpatient Primary Care

A 45 y/o female presents to the office with itching

Vital Signs

Blood pressure: 128/68

Respirations: 12 per minute

Pulse: 76 bpm

Temperature: 98.8°F

Weight: 162 lbs

Height: 5'5"

Pain: 1 out of 10

PATIENT NAME: IZA ICHEN
Clinical Setting: Outpatient Primary Care

Subjective

Objective

Assessment

Plan

CC: A 45 y/o female presents to the office with itching

History

			Performed
	1	Introduces self.	
	2	Explains the role of the provider.	
	3	Opening question: What brings you in today?	I have itching.
Chronology/ Onset	4	When did it **start**?	About a week ago.
	5	Did you ever have this **before**?	Yes.
	6	When was that?	About 2 years ago.
Description	7	**Where do you** itch?	Right between my legs.
Exacerbations	8	Anything make it **worse**?	It itches more when I sweat.
Remittance	9	Anything make it **better**?	Not really.
Symptoms associated	10	Any **vaginal discharge**?	Yes.
	11	What does it **look like**?	It's white, and chunky.
	12	Any **rash**?	Yes, it's really red down there.
	13	**Fever or chills**?	No.
	14	**Burning with urination**?	Just a little bit at the start.
	15	**Polyuria, polydipsia, polyphagia**?	No.
Medical Hx	16	Do you have any other **medical conditions**?	No.
Medications	17	What **medications** are you on?	I just finished a course of antibiotics.
	18	What were you treated for?	Bronchitis.
Allergies	19	Do you have any **allergies**?	Yes, amoxicillin gives me a rash.
Social Hx	20	Are you **sexually active**?	Yes.
	21	**How many partners** do you have?	Just one.
	22	Does your **partner** have any **symptoms**?	No.
	23	Have you ever had an **STD**?	No.
	24	When was the **FDLNMP**?	It's been a couple of months, but I'm never regular.

Physical Exam

	25	Informs patient that the physical exam is to begin.	
	26	Washes hands for 15 seconds.	
Vitals	27	Performs repeat vitals if appropriate.	
General	28	General assessment	Alert, no apparent distress
Neck	29	Palpation of thyroid gland	No thyroidmegaly
Respiratory	30	Auscultation	Clear to auscultation
Cardiac	31	Auscultation: aortic, pulmonic, tricuspid, and mitral	RRR w/o m/r/g

			Performed
Abdominal	32	Inspection	Scaphoid
	33	Auscultation	Normoactive bowel sounds
	34	Palpation	Nontender, without masses
Genital	35	Inspection	Erythematous macular rash vulva
Pelvic	36	Speculum	Thick white exudate with white patches attached to vaginal mucosa Os closed without discharge
	37	Bimanual	Without cervical motion or adnexal tenderness. Normal uterine size.
Assessment/	38	Explained differential diagnosis including vulvovaginitis	
Plan	39	Explained likely etiology: Candidal infection following antibiotic use.	
	40	Explained plan: pregnancy test, urine dip, treatment for candidal infection.	
	41	Asks the patient if she has any questions or suggestions.	
	42	Thanks the patient and offers further assistance.	
	43	Displayed professionalism and empathy throughout the interview.	

Case Review #10

This 45-year-old female presents with vaginal itching of one week duration. She should be asked about the presence of a rash and vaginal discharge. Many board questions are based on the description of vaginal discharge. A history of a white, chunky discharge is classic for vaginal candidiasis. (**BQ**)

It is important to ask if the patient has had yeast infections in the past, and if so, how frequently they occur. Frequent yeast infections should alert to the provider to search for causes of immunodeficiency. Yeast infections are common after taking a course of antibiotics. Diabetes and hypothyroidism can be associated with candidal infections and should be explored on history. You should review the symptoms associated with these two conditions with the patient.

The patient is not experiencing any dysuria, fever, chills, or other urinary symptoms that may have pointed toward a urinary tract infection. Additionally, the patient has not menstruated in several months and pregnancy should be ruled out as it can also be linked with candidal infections. Historically, it is important to assess the patient's risk of having contracted a sexually transmitted disease.

On examination, the patient's thyroid gland should be palpated for enlargement. The pelvic exam confirms a thick white discharge, which points to a candidal infection. There is no cervical motion tenderness, which would point to pelvic inflammatory disease, and no uterine enlargement suggestive of pregnancy.

A pregnancy test should be performed to rule out pregnancy. A urine dip, for glucose in order to rule out possible diabetes, and nitrates in order to rule out a urinary tract infection should also be performed. The patient can then be treated for a candidal infection.

PATIENT NAME: ANITA ENJURIE
Clinical Setting: Family Practice Outpatient Office

A 26 y/o female presents with right knee pain
Vital Signs
Blood pressure: 118/68
Respirations: 12 per minute
Pulse: 72 bpm
Temperature: 98.6°F
Weight: 155 lbs
Height: 5'11"
Pain: 9.5 out of 10

PATIENT NAME: ANITA ENJURIE
Clinical Setting: Family Practice Outpatient Office

Subjective

Objective

Assessment

Plan

CC: A 26 y/o female presents with right knee pain

History

			Performed
	1	Introduces self.	
	2	Explains role of provider.	
	3	Opening question: What brings you in today?	I hurt my knee.
Chronology/ Onset	4	**How** did you hurt it?	Playing football.
	5	**When** did it happen?	Last night at football practice.
	6	Did you hurt this knee **before**?	Yes, last year in basketball.
Description/ Duration	7	**Describe** how it happened.	I was hit on the outside of my knee.
	8	**Where** is the pain?	In my whole knee.
Intensity	9	**Intensity** on a scale of 1 to 10?	A 9.5.
Exacerbation	10	What makes it **worse**?	Standing on it.
Remission	11	What makes it **better**?	Resting it. I put some ice on it, too.
Symptoms associated	12	Any **bruising**?	Yes.
	13	Any **swelling**?	Yes, a lot.
	14	Is the **range of motion** limited?	I can't bend or straighten it the whole way.
	15	Does the knee **click or lock**?	I don't think so.
Medical Hx	16	Do you have any other **medical conditions**?	I have asthma.
	17	What was the **FDLNMP**?	Last week.
Medications	18	What **medications** are you on?	The pill.
Allergies	19	Do you have any **allergies**?	No.
Surgical Hx	20	Any previous **operations**?	Yes.
	21	What was that?	They scoped the same knee.
	22	Did they find anything?	They shaved a little off the meniscus.

Physical Examination

	23	Informs patient that the physical exam is to begin.	
	24	Washes hands for 15 seconds.	
Vitals	25	Correctly performs repeat vitals if appropriate.	
General	26	Assess for **distress from pain**.	Facial grimace present.
MS	27	Assess **gait**.	Limps on right.
	28	Inspection **Expose bilateral** lower extremities and compare:	
	29	**Erythema, ecchymosis, edema**	Diffuse edema of R knee area
	30	Palpation **Compare bilaterally:**	Increased warmth. Tenderness at
	31	**Warmth, tenderness, edema**	medial joint space of R knee

			Performed
32 ROM	**Compare bilaterally**	ROM limited by pain	
33	**Active/passive flexion and extension**	at right knee.	
34 Special tests	**Anterior Drawer—** anterior cruciate ligament laxity	Positive	
35	**Posterior Drawer—** Posterior cruciate ligament laxity	Negative	
36	**Abduction (valgus) stress**—Medial collateral laxity	Positive	
37	**Adduction (varus) stress**—Lateral collateral laxity	Negative	
38	**Patellar tracking—** listen for crepitus	Negative	
39	**Ballottement**—joint effusion	Positive	
40	**McMurray test—** meniscal integrity	Click felt	
Assessment/	41 Give three things in the differential diagnosis including meniscal and ligamental tears.		
Plan	42 Explained plan: imaging, pain control, orthopedic referral.		
	43 Perform appropriate manipulation.		
	44 Asks the patient if she has any questions.		
	45 Thanks the patient. Displayed professionalism and empathy throughout the interview.		

Case Review #11

This is a 26-year-old female who presents with knee pain after a traumatic injury. In cases of traumatic injury, the history portion of the exam is usually straightforward. Past injuries and surgical procedures are important to document.

Additional information should be sought from patients when the injury is out of proportion to the mechanism of action. In these instances, child abuse, domestic violence, or pathologic injuries should be considered.

On physical exam the patient has a positive anterior drawer sign, abduction stress, and McMurray test. This is consistent with the mechanism of action discussed in the history, being hit on the lateral aspect of the knee.

This patient will need pain medications, an MRI to assess the structures of the knee, and an orthopedic referral.

PATIENT NAME: MICHAEL TROOP
Clinical Setting: Urgent Care Center

A 28 y/o Caucasian male presents with back pain

Vital Signs

Blood pressure: 138/85 mmHg

Respirations: 16 per minute

Pulse: 120 bpm

Temperature: 100.8°F

Weight: 162 lbs

Height: 6'1"

Pain: 8 out of 10

PATIENT NAME: MICHAEL TROOP
Clinical Setting: Urgent Care Center

Subjective

Objective

Assessment

Plan

CC: A 28 y/o Caucasian male presents with back pain

History

			Performed
	1	Introduces self.	
	2	Explains role of provider.	
	3	What brings you in today?	My back really hurts.
Chronology/	4	When did it **start**?	About 2 hours ago.
Onset	5	What were you **doing**?	I was grocery shopping.
	6	Did you ever have this **before**?	No.
Description/	7	Was the onset **sudden** or **gradual**?	It was very sudden.
Duration	8	Is the duration **continuous** or does it **come and go**?	It's always there, but sometimes it gets a little better, then bad again.
	9	**Describe** the pain.	Like a huge cramp.
	10	**Where** is the pain?	*Grabs right lateral lumbar area.*
	11	Does it **radiate** anywhere?	It goes down into my right groin.
	12	Where in the groin?	My right ball.
Intensity	13	**Intensity** on a scale of 1 to 10?	A 10.
Exacerbation	14	What makes it **worse**?	I don't think anything.
Remission	15	What makes it **better**?	Nothing.
Symptoms associated	16	Do you have any **burning with urination**?	No.
	17	Do you have any **blood in the urine**?	I haven't seen any.
	18	**Nausea or vomiting**?	I feel like I'm going to vomit.
	19	**Fever or chills**?	Yes, I'm hot and sweaty.
Medical Hx	20	Do you have any other **medical conditions**?	No.
Medications	21	Are you on any **medications**?	Just vitamins.
	22	Which vitamins?	A handful of vitamin C a day.
	23	Why do you do that?	To keep the colds away.
Allergies	24	Do you have any **allergies**?	No.
Social Hx	25	Do you **smoke**?	No.
	26	Do you drink **alcohol**?	A little.
	27	How much do you drink?	One or two beers a week.
Hosp/Surg Hx	28	Have you had any **hospitalizations or surgeries**?	No.

Physical Exam

	29	Informs patient that the physical exam is to begin.
	30	Washes hands for 15 seconds.

			Performed
General	31	Assess for **distress and position of comfort**	Cannot find position of comfort
Vitals	32	Properly performs **repeat vitals if indicated**	
Lungs	33	Auscultation: Instruct patient breathe deeply	Clear to auscultation
	34	Complete inspiration and expiration	
Heart	35	Auscultation: aortic, pulmonic, tricuspid and mitral	Regular rhythm without murmur
Abdomen	36	Inspection **Contour**	Scaphoid
	37	Auscultation **Prior to palpation**	Hyperactive bowel sounds
	38	**All four quadrants**	greatest in the upper quadrants
	39	Palpation: watch the patient's face during palpation	Tenderness in the right lower quadrant. No masses.
	40	**Light and deep**	
	41	Identify **tenderness and masses**	
	42	Percussion **Gas pattern**	Tympanic in the left upper quad
	43	Special tests **Rebound, Rigidity, Guarding**	None
	44	**CVA tenderness**	Positive
Genital	45	Inspection	Normal male genitalia
	46	Palpation	No tenderness, masses, or hernias.
Assessment/ Plan	47	Give three things in the differential diagnosis including nephrolithiasis.	
	48	Explained likely etiology: arrested stone in the urinary system.	
	49	Explained plan: laboratory analysis, UA, X-ray, intravenous fluids, pain management.	
	50	Asks the patient if he has any questions or suggestions.	
	51	Thanks the patient. Displayed professionalism and empathy throughout the interview.	

Case Review #12

This 28-year-old male presents with back pain of sudden onset while shopping. The provider should make sure that there was no recent fall or trauma. He has never had back pain before, which should be confirmed in the past medical and surgical histories. The onset was sudden and is described as cramping in nature.

The key to this diagnosis is the location of the pain, which locates in the right lumbar area and radiates around the flank and into the scrotum. This is a classic (**BQ**) for the presentation of a nephrolithiasis. The patient should be questioned about the symptoms associated with nephrolithiasis including hematuria, dysuria, fever, and nausea. The patient should be asked about a past medical history specifically for kidney stones.

Although the patient does not take prescription medications, he does admit to excessive use of vitamin C. Excess vitamin C precipitates as calcium stones in the urine.

On physical examination, the patient demonstrates an inability to find a position of comfort and he has costovertebral angle tenderness (CVA) to percussion or kidney punch.

True Story

The basis of this case is another true story. When I was in medical school, we had a naturalist physician give us a lecture. He stated he hadn't had a cold in the last 15 years, attributing it to a bowl full of vitamin C that he kept in his kitchen. Whenever he passed by, he would chew up a couple of tablets. It sounded good to me, so I tried the same thing. About a week later, I was shopping with my wife in a local grocery store. She was in another aisle. Suddenly, I had excruciating pain in my back that went down into the scrotum. I started to sweat and felt nauseous. I knew it was a kidney stone and decided to check with a kidney punch on my own. When I hit my own kidney, I nearly passed out. I started down the aisle bent over and holding onto the cart, saying, "find the wife, find the wife!" But by the time I reached the end of the aisle, my pain suddenly vanished. I had passed the stone into my bladder. Now I can truly say that I understand when a patient presents with a stone. (I also tell my students not to overdo the vitamin C.)

NOTES:

PATIENT NAME: JIM ZAHURTIN
Clinical Setting: ER

A 35 y/o Caucasian male presents with abdominal pain
Vital Signs
Blood pressure: 152/98
Respirations: 24 per minute
Temperature: 102°F
Pulse: 92 bpm
Weight: 182 lbs
Height: 5'9"
Pain: 9 out of 10

PATIENT NAME: JIM ZAHURTIN
Clinical Setting: ER

Subjective

Objective

Assessment

Plan

CC: A 35 y/o Caucasian male presents with abdominal pain

History

			Performed
	1	Introduces self.	
	2	Explains role of provider.	
	3	What brings you in today?	My stomach hurts.
Chronology	4	**When** did it **start**?	Last night.
Onset	5	Have you had this **before**?	No.
	6	What were you **doing**?	Getting ready for bed.
	7	Have there been any **changes** in the pain?	It feels like it's moving further down.
Description/	8	**Describe** the pain.	It's sharp and stabbing.
Duration	9	**Constant** or **come and go**?	Constant.
	10	**Where** is it?	Points to RLQ.
	11	Does it **radiate (go)** anywhere?	Sort of into my back.
	12	**Where to**?	*Points to right lumbar region.*
Intensity	13	How severe is it, on a scale from **1 to 10**?	A 9.
Exacerbation	14	What makes it **worse**?	Pushing on my stomach.
Remission	15	Did you try anything to make it **better**?	I tried Tums, but they didn't help.
Symptoms	16	Ask about **nausea or vomiting**?	Once this morning.
associated	17	Any **diarrhea or constipation**?	A little diarrhea this morning.
	18	**Was there any blood or mucus in it**?	No.
	19	Do you **feel hungry**?	No.
	20	**Fever** or **chills**?	I do feel a little warm.
	21	Any **burning** with urination?	No.
Medical Hx	22	Do you have any other **medical conditions**?	I have hypothyroidism.
Medications	23	Are you on any **MEDICATIONS**?	Synthroid.
	24	Do have any **ALLERGIES**?	No.
Allergies	25	Do you **smoke**?	No.
Social Hx	26	Do you **drink**?	Yes.
	27	**How much and how often**?	Two beers once or twice a month.
	28	Do you use any **drugs**?	Just my Synthroid.
Surgical/Hosp	29	Any prior **surgeries** or **hospitalizations**?	No.

Physical Examination

General	30	Assess for **distress**	Moderate pain
	31	**Position of comfort**	Seated flexed at waist

				Performed
Vitals	32	Performs repeat **vital signs** if appropriate		Repeat BP 148/94
HEENT	33	Inspection	Eyes for **icterus**	No icterus
Lungs	34	Auscultation	Instruct patient to **breathe deeply**	Clear to auscultation
	35		**Complete inspiration and expiration**	
Abdomen	36	Inspection	**Contour**	Scaphoid
	37		**Visible pulsations, peristalsis, masses**	None
	38	Auscultation	**prior to palpation**	
	39		**All four quadrants**	
	40		Characterize bowel sounds	Hypoactive
	41	Palpation	**Watch** the patient's **facial expression**	Grimaces with tenderness.
	42		Identify tenderness	Greatest in the RLQ.
	43		**Rebound, Rigidity, Guarding**	Positive
	44		**Masses**	None
	45	Percussion	**Gas pattern**	Results in tenderness.
	46	Special tests	**Rovsing sign**: pain in RLQ with palpation of LLQ	Positive
	47		**Psoas sign**: pain with right thigh extension	Positive
Rectal	48		**Pelvic appendix**: pain at digit and suprapubically	Negative
Assessment	49	Give three things in the differential diagnosis including appendicitis.		
Plan	50	Explained likely etiology: obstruction and inflammation of the appendix.		
	51	Explained plan: CBC, UA, CT scan, surgical consult.		
	52	Asks the patient if he has any questions or suggestions.		
	53	Thanks the patient. Displayed professionalism and empathy.		

Case Review #13

Upon hearing the chief complaint of abdominal pain in a 35-year-old male, your differential diagnosis should minimally include cholecystitis, nephrolithiasis, gastroenteritis, appendicitis, and bowel obstruction. Diverticular disease is less likely because it is usually seen in an older age group.

Your historical questions should be geared at narrowing your differential and determining if the patient has an acute abdomen considered to need surgical intervention.

The patient has a fever, is anorexic, and has had one episode of vomiting and one loose stool. (**BQ**): These historical findings along with the classical presentation of pain, which began periumbilically and has since moved down into the right lower quadrant, suggests acute appendicitis. This emphasizes the need to illicit how the pain has changed since it began.

It is important to ask about prior surgeries. Past surgeries can quickly eliminate a diagnosis from your differential and add others. I once told an ER attendant that the cervix looked fine when the patient had had a total hysterectomy. I really had believed I had seen the cervix but must have seen mucosal folds. A past abdominal surgery may make a bowel obstruction more likely due to adhesions.

The blood pressure is high and should be repeated for accuracy. On exam the bowel sounds are hypoactive and the patient has signs of peritoneal irritation with positive rebound, Rovsing and Psoas signs. The physical signs point to the diagnosis of appendicitis as well.

The plan should include a CBC, UA, CT scan of the abdomen and a surgical consult.

NOTES:

PATIENT NAME: MISSY MENCIES
Clinical Setting: Family Practice Outpatient Office

A 22 y/o female complaining of no menses for three months

Vital Signs

Blood pressure: 110/60

Respirations: 12 per minute

Pulse: 56 bpm

Temperature: 98.4°F

Weight: 110 lbs

Height: 5'4"

Pain: 0 out of 10

PATIENT NAME: MISSY MENCIES
Clinical Setting: Family Practice Outpatient Office

Subjective

Objective

Assessment

Plan

CC: A 22 y/o female is seen in the primary care office c/o no menses for three months

History			Performed
	1	Introduces self.	
	2	Explains role of provider.	
	3	Opening question: What brings you in today?	I haven't had my period.
Chronology/ Onset	4	When was the FDLNMP?	About 4 months ago.
	5	Have you ever missed a period before?	No.
	6	Have your periods changed at all before this?	No.
Obstetric Hx	7	Age at first period?	Thirteen.
	8	Were you regular before this?	Yes.
	9	How many days apart are they normally?	About 25.
	10	How long do they last?	About 5 days.
	11	Describe the flow as heavy, medium, or light.	Two heavy days, and three light.
Sexual Hx	12	Are you sexually active?	Yes.
	13	Do you use protection?	Yes.
	14	What form of protection do you use?	We use the rhythmic cycle.
	15	Have you ever been pregnant?	No.
Symptoms associated	16	Discharge from the breasts?	No.
	17	Symptoms of pregnancy: breast tenderness or enlargement, nausea, vomiting?	They are a little sore.
	18	Symptoms of hypothyroidism: constipation, fatigue, cold intolerance, depression, weight gain, etc.?	No.
	19	Abdominal pain?	No.
	20	Visual changes?	No.
Medical Hx	21	Do you have any other medical conditions?	No.
Medications	22	Are you on any medications?	No.
Social Hx	23	How much do you exercise?	I run 10 miles a day.
	24	How is your diet?	I'm vegetarian.

Performed

Physical Exam

	25	Informs patient that the physical exam is to begin. Has female attendant.	
	26	Washes hands for 15 seconds.	
Vitals	27	Performs repeat vitals if appropriate.	
General	28	General assessment	Alert, timid, no apparent distress
Skin	29	Assess hair texture/pattern, and skin texture	Normal
HEENT	30	Assess for facial hair.	Normal
Neck	31	Palpate the thyroid.	No thyroidmegaly or nodules
Cardiac	32	Auscultation: aortic, pulmonic, tricuspid, and mitral	Normal
Respiratory	33	Auscultation: symmetrical approach	Clear to auscultation
Abdomen	34	Inspection	Slight protuberance infraumbilical
	35	Auscultation	Normal bowel sounds
	36	Percussion	Dullness below the umbilicus
	37	Palpation	Uterine fundus to 18 cm.
Genital	38	Pelvic exam: speculum	Os closed, slight bluish hue
	39	Bimanual	Confirms uterine height
Breast	40	Breasts	Tenderness w/o mass, discharge
Neurologic	41	Visual Fields	Intact
Assessment/	42	Explained differential diagnosis including pregnancy.	
Plan	43	Explained other possible etiologies: exercise induced, etc.	
	44	Explained plan: pregnancy test, other blood work.	
	45	Offer emotional, educational, and medical support.	
	46	Recommend referral to OB/GYN if appropriate.	
	47	Asks the patient if she has any questions.	
	48	Thanks the patient. Displayed professionalism and empathy.	

Case Review #14

This case exemplifies the utility of building a differential diagnosis and efficiently working to confirm your suspicions. When you see that your patient list contains a 22-year-old female who comes to the office because she has not had a menstrual cycle in the past 3 months, your differential diagnosis should minimally include: pregnancy, thyroid dysfunction, exercise induced anovulation, and eating disorders.

In this case, the patient presents complaining of no menses for a precise period of time. If she had not, then one of the first distinctions would be as to whether she had ever had a period, or if she had menstruation in the past but it is no longer occurring; primary amenorrhea or secondary amenorrhea.

It is important to define menarche, the age at first menstruation, if and when the menstrual cycle became regular, how many days apart the menses occur, and how many days it lasts. In addition, it is also important to quantify the amount of bleeding that occurs often categorized as light, moderate, or heavy flow. Often patients will present, not with an absent menses, but with a change from baseline. Specifically asking how the menses has changed is important.

Of course, probably the first and most common diagnosis would be pregnancy. Providers often are hesitant to take a sexual history. Introducing the topic in a nonjudgemental way helps to illicit honest answers. An introductory statement such as, "I have to ask you some questions now that we ask everyone who comes in with a concern like yours. These questions will help us in making the right diagnosis and treatment plan for you," tells the patient that you are not judging them but simply trying to provide the best possible care. This point is emphasized in the male patient who presents with a rectal complaint. At some point after the introduction above, simply asking if anything is ever inserted into the rectum allows the patient to answer as freely as possible.

This patient is sexually active and uses the rhythm method for birth control. In other cases, defining sexual activity may require more explanation. Some people define sexual activity only as having intercourse where penetration occurs. Penetration, however, is not necessary for pregnancy to occur. You may also have to ask if there has been any contact whatsoever with sperm or body fluids. In any case, amenorrhea in females of reproductive age requires evaluation by a pregnancy test.

The symptoms associated provide almost a checklist to prove or disprove the rest of your differential. Here, the patient does not admit to any symptoms associated with hypothyroidism, but she does run 10 miles per day. Dietary habits must also be explored, including those associated with eating disorders.

On physical exam, the patient does not have physical finding suggestive of a thyroid disorder such as thyroidmegaly or hair or skin changes. The patient's uterus is enlarged and the cervix has a bluish hue, both of which are suggestive of pregnancy.

It is important to discuss the patient's feelings toward pregnancy and to provide her with a referral to an OB/GYN should the pregnancy be confirmed.

NOTES:

PATIENT NAME: CHESTER PAINE
Clinical Setting: ER

A 22 y/o male college student with chest pain
Vital Signs
Blood pressure: 180/100
Respirations: 24 per minute
Pulse: 112 bpm
Temperature: 98.8°F
Weight: 190 lbs
Height: 6' 6"
Pain: 8 out of 10

PATIENT NAME: CHESTER PAINE
Clinical Setting: ER

Subjective

Objective

Assessment

Plan

CC: A 22 y/o male college student is brought to the ER with chest pain

History

			Performed
	1 Introduces self.		
	2 Explains role of provider.		
	3 Opening question: What brings you in today?	I have chest pain.	
Chronology/	4 When did it **start**?	About an hour ago.	
Onset	5 What were you **doing**?	Playing basketball.	
	6 Did you ever have this **before**?	No.	
Description/	7 **Describe** the pain.	It's a ripping, a tearing.	
Duration	8 **Where** is the pain?	In the center of my chest.	
	9 Does it radiate anywhere?	Between my shoulder blades.	
	10 Was the onset **sudden** or **gradual**?	It happened all of a sudden.	
	11 Is it **continuous** or does it **come and go**?	Continuous.	
Intensity	12 How would you rate the intensity on a scale of **1 to 10**?	An 8.	
Exacerbation	13 What makes it **worse**?	Nothing.	
Remission	14 What makes it **better**?	Nothing.	
Symptoms	15 Do you feel **lightheaded**?	Yes.	
associated	16 **Nausea or vomiting**?	No.	
	17 **Shortness of breath/cough**?	Yes.	
	18 **Abdominal pain**?	No.	
	19 **Arm or leg pain**?	My right arm.	
	20 **Slurred speech, facial droop**	No.	
	21 **Weakness** or **numbness/tingling**?	No.	
Medical Hx	22 Do you have any other **medical conditions**?	I have Marfan's syndrome.	
Medications	23 What **medications** are you on?	None.	
Allergies	24 Do you have any **allergies**?	No.	
Social Hx	25 Do you **smoke**?	No.	
	26 Do you drink **alcohol**?	No.	
	27 Do you use any **drugs**?	Once in a while.	
	28 What do you use?	A little crack on weekends.	
Surgical/Hosp Hx	29 Have you had any **surgeries** or **hospitalizations**?	No.	

Physical Examination

30	Informs patient that the physical exam is to begin.
31	Washes hands for 15 seconds.

				Performed
Vitals	32	Blood pressure: Compare bilateral upper extremities		R arm 190/110, L 150/100
	33	Pulse—rate and rhythm		Regular at 110 bpm
	34	Respirations—rate		24 bpm
General	35	Assess for distress		Facial grimaces of distress
Neck	36	Assess for JVD		No JVD
Cardiac	37	Inspection	Precordial heave	No heave noted.
	38	Palpation	Locate the PMI	5th ICS MCL
	39	Auscultation	Bell and diaphragm—four valve areas	Grade 1/6 aortic
	40		Identify murmurs	Regurgitant murmur
	41		Identify S1, S2, S3, S4	S1 and S2 without S3, S4
Respiratory	42	Inspection	Cyanosis	None
	43		Accessory muscle use	None
	44	Palpation	Reproducibility of pain with palpation	Not reproducible
	45	Auscultation	Instruct to breathe deeply through the mouth	Clear to auscultation
	46		Complete inspiration and expiration	
Extremities	47	Inspection	Pallor	None
	48	Palpation	Peripheral pulses for symmetry or deficits	3/4 Right arm, 2/4 Left arm
Neurologic	49	Inspection	Cranial nerves II-XII	CN II-XII intact
	50		Strength and comparing bilateral extremities	Equal throughout at 5/5
Assessment	51	Explained differential diagnosis including aortic dissection		
Plan	52	Explained plan: chest X-ray, ECG, CT scan, control blood pressure, stat surgical consult		
	53	Asks the patient if he has any questions.		
	54	Thanks the patient. Displayed professionalism and empathy.		

Case Review #15

Demographics play an important role in developing the differential diagnosis. Here, your patient is a 22-year-old male who presents to the ED complaining of chest pain. Any chest pain case requires consideration of coronary artery disease (CAD), but your suspicion is not as high initially. To expand your differential diagnosis, think of anatomy. In addition to cardiac etiology, your differential diagnosis should include pathology of respiratory, gastrointestinal, musculoskeletal, and psychiatric origin.

Key clues to a quick, accurate assessment include the patient's description of the pain as a tearing sensation in the center of his chest, the location with radiation into the back between the shoulder blades, and the patient's history of Marfan's syndrome. These should alert you to the possibility of an aortic dissection. The tearing quality of the chest pain is a classic Board question in association with a dissecting aortic aneurysm. (**BQ**)

Failing to ask for the past medical history would have left out a major diagnostic clue. Likewise, the social history shows the patient admitting to the use of crack occasionally on the weekends. Cocaine use is more often associated with myocardial infarction, and so, our differential swings between the two.

Symptoms associated focus around those associated with CAD and stroke. Why a stroke? Anatomically, the dissecting aneurysm can extend to include the brachiocephalics producing extremity pain due to poor perfusion, or stroke symptoms such as slurred speech, facial droop, or extremity weakness, and paresthesia if cerebral perfusion is affected.

On physical exam, the blood pressure should be repeated in both arms along with palpation of the pulses, again assessing extension of the dissection. The difference in the BP between the left and right arms and asymmetrical peripheral pulses in the upper extremity is common in aortic dissection due to the partial blockage of the subclavian arteries.

Assess for signs of heart failure such as jugular venous distension (JVD) and crackles. This patient has an aortic regurgitant murmur, which can be seen in cases of proximal dissection.

The patient's cranial nerves and strength testing are intact, which makes cerebral compromise less likely.

Time is of the essence in this patient. The plan should include stat chest imaging, an ECG, blood pressure control, and a cardiovascular surgical consult.

NOTES:

PATIENT NAME: MIA C. FALGIA
Clinical Setting: Family Practice Outpatient Office Visit

A 22 y/o female presents with a headache

Vital Signs

Blood pressure: 110/60

Respirations: 16 per minute

Pulse: 72 bpm

Temperature: 98.0°F

Weight: 128 lbs

Height: 5' 4"

Pain: 7 out of 10

PATIENT NAME: MIA C. FALGIA
Clinical Setting: Family Practice Outpatient Office Visit

Subjective

Objective

Assessment

Plan

CC: A 22 y/o female presents with a headache

History

			Performed
	1	Introduces self.	
	2	Explains role of provider.	
	3	Opening question: What brings you in today?	I have a headache.
Chronology/	4	When did it **start**?	Well, this one started about 2 days ago.
Onset	5	Was the onset **sudden** or **gradual**?	They come on gradually.
	6	**How often** do they occur?	I use to get them once a month, now I get one once a week.
	7	When did you **first start getting them**?	About 2–3 years ago.
	8	Can you tell they are **coming on**?	I see a fuzzy bright spot which gets bigger and bigger. Then the headache starts.
	9	What are you **doing at onset**?	They can happen any time.
	10	**Triggers**? (foods, stress, fatigue)	Not that I know of.
Description	11	**Describe** the headaches.	It's a pounding in my head.
	12	**Location**?	They're always on the right side.
Intensity	13	Scale of **1 to 10**?	They can go up to a 10.
Exacerbation	14	What makes the headache **worse**?	Bright lights.
Remission	15	What makes the headache **better**?	I take ibuprofen and go to bed.
Symptoms associated	16	**Nausea**?	Yes, after it starts, I feel like I want to vomit.
	17	**Numbness/tingling/weakness**?	No.
	18	**Depression or anxiety**?	Only about these headaches.
	19	**Fever or chills**?	No.
	20	**Tooth, ear, or sinus pain**?	No.
Medical Hx	21	Do you have any other **medical conditions**?	No.
	22	History of **head trauma**?	No.
Medications	23	What **medications** are you on?	None.
Allergies	24	Do you have any **allergies**?	No.
Social Hx	25	Do you **smoke, drink alcohol, or use any drugs**?	No.
Surgical/Hosp	26	Have you had any **surgeries** or hospitalizations?	No.
FDLNMP	27	When was the FDLNMP?	A week or two ago.

Performed

Physical Exam

	28	Informs patient that the physical exam is to begin.	
	29	Washes hands for 15 seconds.	
Vitals	30	Performs repeat vitals if appropriate.	
General	31	General assessment	Alert, no apparent distress
Head	32	Inspection, palpation	NCAT, nontender to palpation
Sinuses	33	Palpation, percussion	Nontender
Eyes	34	Ophthalmoscopic examination	Cup:disc ratio 1:2 with sharp margin
Nose	35	Inspection	No exudate, edema, masses
Ears	36	Inspection	TMs gray bilaterally
Mouth/throat	37	Inspection	Teeth in good repair, no lesions, moist
Neck	38	Inspection, palpation	Symmetrical, no masses, non-tender to palp
			Tissue texture changes T1-4 Right
Cardiac	39	Auscultation: aortic, pulmonic, tricuspid, and mitral	RR w/o murmur, rub, or gallop
Respiratory	40	Auscultation: symmetrical approach	Clear to auscultation
Neurologic	41	**Cranial nerves**: performs II-XII assessment	Intact
	42	**Muscle strength**	5/5 throughout
	43	**Reflexes**: bilateral upper and lower extremities	2/4 throughout
Assessment/	44	Give three things in the differential diagnosis including migraine.	
Plan	45	Explained plan: medication, manipulation, consider CT scan, identifying triggers.	
	46	Performs appropriate manipulation.	
	47	Asks the patient and family if they have any questions.	
	48	Thanks the patient. Displayed professionalism and empathy.	

Case Review #16

This 22-year-old female presents to the office with a headache. The majority of headaches are benign. It is important to rule out a secondary cause of headache, which could be life-threatening. A thorough history is important. The majority of headaches are diagnosed through historical data because most patients do not have any physical findings.

Headache caused by an infection (tooth, ear, or sinus), stress, head trauma and migraine should be included in your differential diagnosis. Poor dental hygiene is one of the most common causes of facial pain.

This patient has a past history of similar headaches. The headaches have an aura (a fuzzy bright spot that gets bigger and bigger.) Bright lights make the headache worse and they are relieved with sleep, which points to the diagnosis of migraine.

An important consideration is that this patient's headaches have become more frequent. There is a change in the headache pattern. If the patient hadn't volunteered that the headaches were becoming more frequent, an appropriate question would have been, "How have the headaches changed?"

On physical examination, infection should be ruled out by checking the sinuses, nose, ears, mouth, and throat. A funduscopic exam should be performed to rule out papilledema. If a patient has papilledema, nuchal rigidity or a focal defect on cranial nerve exam, then a CT scan should be performed immediately. These findings point to a secondary cause of the headache.

If there is no papilledema, nuchal rigidity or focal defects on neurological exam, then the decision to order a CT is made based on clinical judgment. This patient has had a change in her headache pattern. The headaches are occurring on a more frequent basis, so this may warrant a CT scan.

Treatment options for this patient would include the possibility of starting daily medication to prevent her headaches instead of waiting for the headache to occur and then treating the symptoms.

Manipulation can be performed and the patient should try to identify any triggers that lead to a headache in order to avoid them.

NOTES:

PATIENT NAME: GALE MASON
Clinical Setting: Family Practice Outpatient Office

A 43 y/o Caucasian female presents for abdominal pain
Vital Signs
Blood pressure: 138/85
Respirations: 16 per minute
Pulse: 80 bpm
Temperature: 100.8°F
Weight: 189 lbs
Height: 5'4"
Pain: 8 out of 10

PATIENT NAME: GALE MASON
Clinical Setting: Family Practice Outpatient Office

Subjective

Objective

Assessment

Plan

CC: A 43 y/o Caucasian female presents for abdominal pain

History

			Performed
	1	Introduces self.	
	2	Explains the role of the provider.	
	3	What brings you in today?	My stomach hurts.
Chronology/	4	When did it **start**?	Last night.
Onset	5	What were you **doing**?	Just sitting at home.
	6	Did you ever have this **before**?	Yes.
	7	When?	On and off for about 6 months.
Description/	8	Was the onset **sudden** or **gradual**?	Gradual.
Duration	9	Is the duration **continuous** or does it **come and go**?	Continuous since last night.
	10	**Describe** the pain.	Like a cramping.
	11	**Where** is the pain?	*Points to right upper quadrant.*
	12	Does it **radiate** anywhere?	Kind of goes into my back.
	13	Where in the back?	*Points to right scapula.*
Intensity	14	**Intensity** on a scale of 1 to 10?	An 8.
Exacerbation	15	What makes it **worse**?	Eating.
Remission	16	What makes it **better**?	Nothing.
Symptoms	17	Do you have any **heartburn**?	Sometimes.
associated	18	**Nausea** or **vomiting**?	I feel like vomiting.
	19	**Diarrhea** or **constipation**?	No.
	20	**Fever** or **chills**?	I feel hot when I get the pain.
	21	**Difficulty breathing** or **cough**?	No.
Medical Hx	22	Do you have any other **medical conditions**?	I just had a baby last year.
Medications	23	Are you on any **medications**?	Just birth control pills.
Allergies	24	Do you have any **allergies**?	No.
Social Hx	25	Do you **smoke**?	No.
	26	Do you drink **alcohol**?	A little.
	27	How **much** do you drink?	A glass of wine once a month.
Hosp/Surg Hx	28	Have you had any **hospitalizations** or **surgeries**?	I had a C-section.
Menstrual Hx	29	When was the **FDLNMP**?	I haven't had one since I had the baby.

Physical Exam

	30	Informs patient that the physical exam is to begin.
	31	Washes hands for 15 seconds.

Performed

Section	#	Task		Finding
General	32	Assess for **distress and position of comfort**		Flexes toward and holds RUQ
Vitals	33	Properly performs **repeat vitals if indicated**.		
HEENT	34	Inspection	Eyes for icterus	No icterus
Lungs	35	Auscultation	Instructs the patient to **breathe deeply**	Faint crackles in RLL otherwise clear to auscultation
	36		**Complete inspiration and expiration**	
Heart	37	Auscultation:	Aortic, pulmonic, tricuspid, and mitral	Regular rhythm without murmur
Abdomen	38	Inspection	**Contour**	Moderately obese
	39		Visible **pulsations or peristalsis**	None
	40	Auscultation	**Prior to palpation All four quadrants**	Hyperactive bowel sounds greatest in the upper quadrants
	41	Palpation:	Watch the patient's face during palpation	Patient grimaces with palpation of epigastria.
			Light and deep identify **tenderness**	No masses.
	42	Percussion	**Gas pattern**	Tympanic in the left upper quad
	43	Special tests	**Rebound, Rigidity, Guarding**	Guarding of the epigastria
	44		**Murphy exam**	Positive
Rectal	45		**Hemoccult**	Negative
Assessment/	46	Give three things in the differential diagnosis including cholelithiasis.		
Plan	47	Explained likely etiology: obstruction and inflammation of the gallbladder.		
	48	Explained plan: laboratory analysis, UA, ultrasound, antibiotics, surgical consult.		
	49	Asks the patient if she has any questions or suggestions.		
	50	Thanks the patient. Displayed professionalism and empathy.		

Case Review #17

This is a 43-year-old female who presents to the office complaining of abdominal pain. Upon hearing the chief complaint, your differential diagnosis is quite broad, encompassing at least the gastrointestinal and genitourinary systems. Your historical questions should be geared at narrowing your differential and determining if the patient has an acute abdomen.

The patient has had similar episodes for the past 6 months. The pain is in the right upper quadrant (RUQ), radiates to her scapula (BQ) and is described as crampy. Use the anatomical location as a guide to your diagnosis. What anatomically lies in the RUQ? Start anteriorly and work posteriorly. Does the patient have a skin rash suggestive of zoster? Does movement make it worse or has she had any trauma suggesting musculoskeletal origin? Does she have diarrhea associated with colitis? Has she had dyspepsia suggestive of gastric or duodenal ulceration? Has she noticed yellowness in her eyes, a sign of gall stones? Think of each organ system encountered and ask the appropriate question to rule in or out the associated diagnosis.

Here, the patient admits to an association with eating and nausea. These historical findings along with pain in the RUQ suggest cholecystitis or ulceration.

It is important to ask about prior surgeries. Past surgeries can quickly eliminate a diagnosis from your differential. A past abdominal surgery may make a bowel obstruction more likely.

On examination, notate the patient's position of comfort. Begin the exam from head to toe but with a problem-specific focus. Many providers skip the examination of the sclera, the first place hyperbilirubinemia will be noticed with bile duct obstruction. The bowel sounds are hyperactive and the patient has a positive Murphy sign. The physical signs point to the diagnosis of cholelithiasis.

Think of the 5 Fs: female, fat, forty, fertile, and flatulence. (Perhaps we should use the word "fluffy" instead of fat.)

The plan should include a CBC, UA, ultrasound, antibiotics, and a surgical consult. Don't forget the pregnancy test.

NOTES:

PATIENT NAME: D. LOU SHUNEL
Clinical Setting: Primary Care Office

A 21 y/o male is brought into your office by his mother, who believes he is on drugs

Vital Signs

Blood pressure: 120/72

Respirations: 16 per minute

Pulse: 92 bpm

Temperature: 98.8°F

Weight: 160 lbs

Height: 6'1"

Pain: 0 out of 10

PATIENT NAME: D. LOU SHUNEL
Clinical Setting: Primary Care Office

Subjective

Objective

Assessment

Plan

CC: A 21 y/o male is brought into your office by his mother, who believes he is on drugs

(Patient's answers are in regular type. Mother's answers are in bold-faced type.)

History			Performed
	1	Introduces self.	
	2	Explains role of provider.	
	3	Opening question: What brings you in today?	You know why. I heard you on the phone and saw you in the TV.
Chronology/	4	**When was that?**	You know. **It started about a year ago.**
Onset	5	How has it **changed?**	**It's all the time now.**
	6	Did this ever have this **before?**	I know you're in with them. I see them.
Description	7	**Describe** what's been happening.	**He thinks everyone is out to get him.**
Intensity	8	Effect on **Activity of Daily Living?**	**He won't leave the house.**
Exacerbations	9	Does anything make this **worse?**	No.
Remitting factors	10	Does anything make this **better?**	No.
Symptoms	11	Do you ever **hear voices?**	Do I ever NOT hear voices?
associated	12	What do the voices say?	You know. You can hear them too.
			And I'll be the king forever.
			Riding the waves.
	13	Any history of **trauma/head injury?**	No.
	14	**Anxiety?**	**He seems jumpy.**
	15	**Depression?**	**He can be really monotone.**
	16	**Thoughts of hurting yourself or others?**	They want me. I'll fight.
	17	**Fever or chills?**	Fire burns, water heals.
	18	**Weight loss or gain?**	Eat the poison yourself, bug man.
Medical Hx	19	Do you have any other **medical conditions?**	No.
Medications	20	Do you take any **medications?**	No.
Allergies	21	Do you have any **allergies?**	No.
Social Hx	22	Do you **smoke?**	No.
	23	Do you drink **alcohol?**	No.
	24	Do you use any **drugs?**	**He must be on something.** **He has to be.** Drug, bug, drug the bug.
Surg/Hosp Hx	25	Any **surgeries** or **hospitalizations?**	No.

Performed

Family Hx	26	Family member w/hx of mental illness?	**My brother disappeared at his age.**
Physical Exam			
	27	Informs patient that the physical exam is to begin.	
	28	Washes hands for 15 seconds.	
Vitals	29	Performs repeat vitals properly if appropriate.	
General	30	General assessment	Alert, NAD, unkempt.
HEENT	31	Inspection	NCAT
			Will not allow exam of the mouth.
Neck	32	Inspection for symmetry, masses, thyroidmegaly	Symmetrical without masses
	33	Palpation for masses, thyroidmegaly	Refuses palpation.
Cardiac	34	Auscultation: aortic, pulmonic, tricuspid, and mitral	RR w/o murmur, rub, or gallop
Respiratory	35	Auscultation: symmetrical approach	Clear to auscultation
Neurologic	36	Cranial nerves: performs II-XII assessment	II-XII intact
	37	Muscle strength: B/l upper and lower extremities	5/5 throughout
	38	Sensation	Becomes defensive at sight of safety pin.
	39	Reflexes	Becomes defensive at sight of hammer.
	40	Cerebellar examination: finger nose, heal shin, rapid alternating movements	Will not cooperate.
Mental Status	41	Orientation	Alert to person, place and time.
Assessment/	42	Explained differential diagnosis including schizophrenia.	
Plan	43	Explained likely etiology and prognosis: Unknown cause, chronic disorder.	
	44	Explained plan: psych consult, CT scan, CBC, chem, TSH, folic acid, B_{12}, VDRL, drug screen	
	45	Asks the patient and family if they have any questions.	
	46	Thanks the patient. Displayed professionalism and empathy throughout the interview.	

Case Review #18

This is a 21-year-old male who is brought into the office by his mother because she thinks that he is on drugs. Drug use should be part of the differential diagnosis; however, medical causes for changes in personality or behavior must not be overlooked.

Upon questioning the patient, it is apparent that the patient is delusional, paranoid, and socially withdrawn. Much of the accurate history is obtained only from his mother. It is important to define which behaviors he is exhibiting that makes her believe that he is using drugs.

The onset of psychotic symptom in schizophrenia commonly occurs in the twenties, placing the patient in the correct age group. Assure that there has been no recent trauma. Ask if drug use or drug paraphernalia has been observed or if the patient has had prior arrests or problems related to drug use.

Despite the confusing answers obtained from the patient, the same basic questioning proves fruitful. Providers should not allow themselves to be distracted from their goals. If you become lost, fall back on mnemonic.

The family history shows that an uncle disappeared at the age of 21. There may be a history of schizophrenia in the family.

The physical exam should be geared at ruling out a secondary cause of psychosis. A neurological exam is done to evaluate the patient for loss of fine motor movements common in schizophrenia. This patient is uncooperative with many aspects of the examination and should not be forced to participate.

The plan should include a psychiatric consult, a CT scan, and laboratory diagnostic exams to rule out a secondary cause of the psychosis such as a thyroid disorder, syphilis, vitamin deficiency, and drug abuse. An urgent inpatient admission may be warranted.

NOTES:

PATIENT NAME: GRAHAM KRACKER
Clinical Setting: ER

A 62 y/o Caucasian male presents to the ER with chest pain

Vital Signs

Blood pressure: 180/104

Respirations: 20 per minute

Pulse: 108 bpm

Temperature: 99.2°F

Weight: 210 lbs

Height: 6'1"

Pain: 8 out of 10

PATIENT NAME: GRAHAM KRACKER
Clinical Setting: ER

Subjective

Objective

Assessment

Plan

CC: A 62 y/o Caucasian male presents to the ER with chest pain

			Performed
HPI:	1	Introduces self.	
	2	Explains role of provider.	
	3	Opening question: What brings you in today?	I was having chest pain.
Chronology/ Onset	4	When did it **start**?	An hour ago.
	5	What were you **doing when it started**?	Walking around the hospital.
	6	Was the onset **sudden** or **gradual**?	Sudden.
	7	Did you ever have this **before**?	Yes.
	8	When?	All last year, whenever I walk my dogs.
	9	Have you ever had this pain at rest?	Just in the past couple months.
Description/ Duration	10	How long does the pain **last**?	Usually 3 to 4 minutes.
	11	How has it **changed**?	I can't walk as far before I get the pain.
	12	How far can you walk now?	Two blocks.
	13	**Describe** the pain.	Sharp, aching, deep.
	14	**Where** is the pain?	*Points just above the xiphoid process.*
	15	Does it radiate anywhere?	No.
Intensity	16	Rate the **intensity** on a scale of 1 to 10?	A 7 or 8.
Exacerbation	17	What makes it **worse**?	Walking.
Remission	18	What makes it **better**?	Resting for a few minutes.
Symptoms associated	19	Was there any **sweating** associated with it?	Sometimes, but just on my face.
	20	Do you have any **nausea** or **vomiting**?	Sometimes a little nausea.
	21	**Shortness of breath**?	Only a little, with the pain.
	22	**Dyspepsia**?	No.
	23	**Cough**?	No.
Medical Hx	24	Medical conditions (HTN, hyperlipidemia, DM)?	High blood pressure and hyperlipidemia.
Medications	25	What **medications** are you on?	Hydrochlorothiazide and Lovastatin.
Allergies	26	Do you have any **allergies**?	No.
Social Hx	27	Do you **smoke**?	Yes.

				Performed
	28	How much do you smoke a day?		Two packs a day.
	29	How long have you been smoking?		Twenty-five years.
	30	Do you drink **alcohol**?		Yes.
	31	How many drinks a day?		2–3 beers a day.
	32	Do you use any **drugs**?		No.
Family Hx	33	Family with early **heart attack or stroke**?		My parents had heart attacks in their 50s.
Physical Examination				
	34	Informs patient that the physical exam is to begin.		
	35	Washes hands for 15 seconds.		
Vitals	36	Correctly performs vital signs.		BP 150/92, P-96 reg, R-20
General	37	Assess for **distress**		No respiratory distress
Neck	38	Assess for **JVD**		No JVD
Cardiac	39	Inspection: **Precordial heave**		No heave
	40	Palpation: Locate the PMI		Anterior axillary line 5th ICS
	41	Auscultation: **Four areas** (aortic, pulmonic, tricuspid, and mitral)		
	42		With **diaphragm and bell**	
	43		Identify **S1 and S2**	Normal S1 and S2
	44		Identify **murmurs, S3 and S4**	No murmurs, S3 or S4
Respiratory	45	Inspection:	**Labor, cyanosis, access muscle use**	No respiratory distress
	46	Palpation: Reproducibility of **pain with palpation**		No tenderness
	47	Auscultation: **Instruct the patient to breathe deeply through the mouth**		
	48		Thorough **complete inspiration and expiration**	Clear to auscultation
	49		Identify **rhonchi, wheezes, crackles**	
Abdomen	50	Inspection: **pulsations**		No pulsations
	51	Palpation: pulsatile masses		No masses
Extremities	52	Inspection: edema		No edema

		Performed
Assessment	53 Give three things in the differential diagnosis including unstable angina.	
Plan	54 Explained plan: stat chest X-ray, ECG, cardiac profile, aspirin, beta-blocker.	
	55 Explained pathophysiology: abnormality in perfusion of the heart.	
	56 Asks the patient if he has any questions.	
	57 Thanks the patient. Displayed professionalism and empathy throughout the interview.	

Case Review #19

When assessing the complaint of chest pain, development of a time line for onset of symptoms not only aids in diagnosis, but also guides appropriate treatment. This patient gives a rather classic presentation of angina with pain on exertion. To distinguish between stable and unstable angina, one must ask about increasing frequency or pain with rest, which by definition is unstable angina. Stable angina occurs with exertion and resolves with rest.

Chest pain associated with coronary artery disease classically has the description of squeezing, pressure, or the feeling that "someone is sitting on my chest." This describes parasympathetic or visceral pain as apposed to sharp, stabbing pain that is more often sympathetic or musculoskeletal in nature. The patient may also place a clenched fist over the left chest. Musculoskeletal pain in comparison is often described as sharp and stabbing. This pain is often made worse by movement, cough, and a deep breath, or by pushing on the area.

In this case, the patient gave himself an impromptu stress test. He had been having chest pain each time he walked his dogs. His primary provider had arranged an exercise stress test in the upcoming week. On the day he presented to the ER, he had been at the hospital for blood work and decided to do a few laps around the hospital to bring out the pain, and he was successful.

It is important to determine the patient's risk for coronary artery disease through historical questions. The patient is male and on medications for high blood pressure and hyperlipidemia. He smokes and has a family history of heart disease. The family history of early cardiovascular disease should be defined as occurring in a family member when they were in their fifties, or younger. The remaining question to ask would include specific past medical history.

Repeat vital signs should be obtained. On physical exam the patient's level of discomfort should be noted. The patient should be assessed for signs of heart failure (JVD, S3, crackles in the lungs and edema), an enlarged heart by locating the PMI, and valvular disease. The chest examination should include pressing on the chest to see if the pain is reproducible.

This patient's historical and physical findings point to pain of a cardiac origin. His pain had resolved but the standard of care still suggests a chest pain protocol should be followed. He should be given an aspirin and started on a beta-blocker. The patient should have a stat chest X-ray to rule out a widened mediastinum, ECG to be read within 10 minutes of arrival, and a cardiac profile. Based on these studies, he may require thrombolytics or a cardiac catheterization.

NOTES:

PATIENT NAME: FRED TRAIN
Clinical Setting: Primary Care Office

A 42 y/o obese male complains of excessive fatigue

Vital Signs

Blood pressure: 165/98

Respirations: 16 per minute

Pulse: 62 bpm

Temperature: 98°F

Weight: 355 lbs

Height: 5'11"

Pain: 0 out of 10

PATIENT NAME: FRED TRAIN
Clinical Setting: Primary Care Office

Subjective

Objective

Assessment

Plan

CC: A 42 y/o obese male complains of excessive fatigue

History			Performed
	1	Introduces self.	
	2	Explains role of provider.	
	3	Opening question: What brings you in today?	I can't keep my eyes open. I fall asleep at work. I'm going to lose my job.
Chronology/ Onset	4	**When** did this start?	Oh, it's been years, Doc.
	5	How has it **changed**?	I fall asleep 3 or 4 times a day.
	6	Did this ever have this **before**?	Like I said, for the last couple of years.
Description	7	**Describe** what's been happening.	I'm just tired.
Intensity	8	Have you ever fallen asleep while driving?	No.
Exacerbations	9	Does anything make this **worse**?	No.
Remissions	10	Does anything make this **better**?	No.
Symptoms associated	11	Do you **snore**?	My wife says I do. She sleeps in another room mostly.
	12	Do you **wake yourself up**?	Yeah, quite a bit.
	13	How do you **sleep at night**?	I just don't feel rested when I get up.
	14	Any problems **concentrating**?	Yeah, I can never finish a TV show.
	15	**Depression**?	Yeah, I'm down, but wouldn't you be?
	16	**Anxiety** or panic attacks?	No.
	17	**Heartburn**?	No.
Medical Hx	18	Do you have any other **medical conditions**?	High blood pressure and low thyroid.
	19	**History of seizures**?	No.
Medications	20	What **medications** are you on?	Atenolol and Synthroid.
Allergies	21	Do you have any **allergies**?	No.
Social Hx	22	Do you **smoke**?	No.
	23	Do you drink **alcohol**?	I have a couple of beers a night.
	24	Do you use any **drugs**?	No.
Surg/Hosp Hx	25	**Surgeries** or hospitalizations?	I'm thinking of that stomach surgery.

Performed

Physical Exam

			Performed
	26	Informs patient that the physical exam is to begin.	
	27	Washes hands for 15 seconds.	
Vitals	28	Perform repeat vitals if appropriate.	BP 162/96
General	29	General assessment	Fatigued appearance, obese.
HEENT	30	Inspection	Infraorbital venous pooling.
			Edentulous.
Neck	31	Inspection	Symmetrical without masses.
	32	Palpation	No masses or thyroidmegaly.
Cardiac	33	Auscultation: aortic, pulmonic, tricuspid, mitral	Distant, RR without murmur.
Respiratory	34	Auscultation: symmetrical approach	Distant but clear to auscultation
Abdomen	35	Inspection, auscultation, palpation order	Obese, hypoactive bowel sounds
Neurologic	36	Orientation	Alert and oriented: person, place and time
	37	**Cranial nerves**: performs II-XII assessment	II-XII intact
	38	**Muscle strength:**	5/5 throughout
	39	**Reflexes**: bilateral upper and lower extremities	1/4 throughout
Assessment/	40	Explained differential diagnosis including sleep apnea.	
Plan	41	Explained likely etiology: airway obstruction likely related to obesity.	
	42	Explained plan: sleep apnea study for CPAP indication, possible surgical intervention, weight loss.	
	43	Asks the patient and family if they have any questions.	
	44	Thanks the patient and offers further assistance.	
	45	Displayed professionalism and empathy throughout the interview.	

Case Review #20

This is a 42-year-old male presenting to the office complaining of excessive fatigue. Your differential diagnosis may initially include sleep apnea, hypothyroidism, narcolepsy, anemia, and inadequate sleep time.

This patient is obese and has a history of HTN and hypothyroidism. He states that he snores so loudly that his wife usually sleeps in another room. He is having difficulty concentrating at work and admits to feeling depressed.

The patient should be questioned regarding falling asleep while driving. If the patient admits to having a hard time staying awake while driving, the practitioner has an obligation to inform the department of motor vehicles. Other sleep-related questions may include likelihood of falling asleep in certain situations such as after meals, while talking with others, and while watching television.

The patient denies a history of anxiety and panic disorder. The patient has a known history of hypothyroidism. Compliance with mediations should be ascertained. If he is compliant, perhaps his current dosing of thyroid medication is subtherapeutic. Medications can also be causative agents of fatigue. This patient is on a beta-blocker. After completing the history, sleep apnea appears to be a likely diagnosis.

On physical exam, the patient's BP should be repeated as the initial screening was high. The patient is not at goal for HTN and the practitioner should consider an adjustment in the patient's medication. He should return to the office within the next month for a repeat BP check.

The patient appears fatigued and has sluggish reflexes throughout. Otherwise the physical exam is benign. The oral pharynx should be examined for evidence of erythema, large tonsils, and uvular excessive soft tissue and a prominent tongue, which are associated with sleep apnea. Heart and lung sound are distant, which is a result of the patient's obesity.

The patient should be evaluated for sleep apnea. Prior to the patient leaving the office, he should be educated on sleep apnea and the need for lifestyle modifications. The patient should advised to follow a low sodium, low fat diet and limit his alcohol intake. Alcohol should not be ingested close to bedtime. Exercise should be encouraged.

NOTES:

PATIENT NAME: IVA KAUFFMAN
Clinical Setting: Family Practice Outpatient Office

A 70 y/o Caucasian female presents with a cough

Vital Signs

Blood pressure: 110/50

Respirations: 24 per minute

Pulse: 112 bpm

Temperature: 101°F

Weight: 160 lbs

Height: 5'2"

Pain: 0 out of 10

PATIENT NAME: IVA KAUFFMAN
Clinical Setting: Family Practice Outpatient Office

Subjective

Objective

Assessment

Plan

CC: A 70 y/o Caucasian female presents to the office with a cough

History			Performed
	1	Introduces self.	
	2	Explains role of provider.	
	3	Opening question: What brings you in today?	I have a cough.
Chronology/	4	When did it **start**?	About a week ago.
Onset	5	How has it **changed** since then?	It keeps me up at night now.
Description/	6	Did you ever have this **before**?	No.
Duration	7	Did it come on **suddenly or gradually**?	Gradually.
	8	**Describe** the cough.	It's wet.
	9	Are you **bringing up** anything?	Yes.
	10	What color is it?	White or yellow.
	11	Does it have any blood in it?	No.
Exacerbation	12	Does anything make it **worse**?	It seems worse in the evening.
Remission	13	Did you try anything to make it **better**?	Cough medicine hasn't helped.
Symptoms	14	Any **runny nose**?	Yes.
associated	15	What color is the nasal drainage?	Clear.
	16	**Post-nasal drainage**?	Not really.
	17	**Sore throat**?	Maybe a little.
	18	**Shortness of breath and dyspnea on exertion**?	I get winded going to the kitchen.
	19	**Fever** or **chills**?	No.
	20	**Night sweats** or **weight loss**?	No.
	21	**Wheezing**?	I don't think so.
	22	**Chest pain**?	Just when I cough.
	23	**Shortness of breath when you are lying flat**?	Yes, I sleep in the recliner.
Medical Hx	24	Do you have any other **medical conditions**?	High blood pressure.
Medications	25	What **medications** are you on?	Some new blood pressure pill.
Allergies	26	Do you have any **allergies**?	No.
Social Hx	27	Do you **smoke**?	Yes.
	28	How much do you smoke a day?	One pack a day.
	29	How long have you been smoking?	Fifty years.

Performed

Physical Examination

	30	Informs patient that the physical exam is to begin.	
	31	Washes hands for 15 seconds.	
Vitals	32	Correctly preforms vitals.	Pulse 112 reg
General	33	Assess for **distress**	No respiratory distress
Skin	34	Assess for **cyanosis**	No cyanosis
HEENT	35	Assess for **nasal mucosa edema and exudate**	Pink without exudate
	36	Assess for **sinus pressure and transillumination**	No tenderness
	37	Assess for **pharyngeal erythema, exudate, PND**	Pink without lesions or exudate
Neck	38	Assess for **JVD**	3 cm JVD
	39	Palpate for **lymphadenopathy** in all nodal areas	No lymphadenopathy
Lungs	40	Inspection **Accessory muscle use**	Mild accessory muscle use
	41	Palpation **Symmetrical rise and fall**	Symmetrical rise and fall
	42	Auscultation Instruct the patient to **breathe deeply through the mouth**	
	43	Complete inspiration and expiration	
	44	Identify adventitious sounds: wheezes, crackles	Crackles bilateral lower lobes
	45	Identify decreased breath sounds	Diminished basilar breath sounds
Heart	46	Auscultation At **aortic, pulmonic, tricuspid, and mitral areas**	
	47	Identify **murmurs**	No murmur
	48	Identify **S1, S2, S3, and S4**	S3
Extremities	49	Inspection/palpation: **Edema**	2+ peripheral edema
	50	Explained differential diagnosis including congestive heart failure.	
	51	Explained plan: chest X-ray, ECG, diuresis, CBC, chemistry panel, ACE inhibitor.	
	52	Asks the patient if she has any questions.	
	53	Thanks the patient. Displayed professionalism and empathy.	

Case Review #21

Previewing the face sheet, we see that the patient complains of a cough and has a fever with tachycardia bringing the pulmonary and cardiac systems to the forefront.

This patient has a cough that began one week ago and is now keeping her up at night. Again, there are many questions that could be asked but that are not included in the Flows. Specifically asking "what" is keeping the patient up would refine your diagnosis. Is the patient being kept awake simply because of a tickle in the throat, or is it because she feels that she cannot get enough oxygen?

Questioning should be geared at determining if the cough is a result of an infection or if it has a cardiac cause. The provider should ask if the cough is productive and, if so, what the sputum looks like and if it contains blood. For instance, rust colored sputum is associated with streptococcal pneumonia. (**BQ**)

The patient now becomes short of breath walking to the kitchen (dyspnea on exertion) and she sleeps in a recliner (orthopnea and PND). Acute precipitations of congestive heart failure (CHF) are often caused by pulmonary infections or medications such as calcium channel blockers. In this patient's case it would be important to determine what new BP medication she has recently started. Angiotensin converting enzyme inhibitors (ACEI) may cause a persistent dry cough.

The patient should also be questioned about chest pain. If the patient has had a recent MI the damage to heart may be the cause of the patient's heart failure.

On physical examination, the patient's pulse should be rechecked noting tachycardia on the face sheet. Determine if she has a dysrhythmia such as atrial fibrillation which has caused her to go into heart failure. Note her general appearance to assure that there is no acute respiratory distress.

With the complaint of rhinorrhea, a limited HEENT exam identifying signs of an upper respiratory tract infection would be appropriate. The majority of your exam, however, should focus on the pulmonary and cardiac system.

Her history of orthopnea and dyspnea on exertion (DOE) pushes you toward congestive heart failure. The exam should focus on the signs commonly associated. She has 3 cm jugular venous distention (JVD), crackles at the bases of her lungs, an S3, and peripheral edema. All of these symptoms point to heart failure.

Heart failure is a symptom. The etiology is still to be found. Your plan should include: an ECG to rule out dysrhythmia, hypertrophy, and MI; a CBC to rule out infection and anemia; chemistry panel to evaluate BUN, creatine, and liver enzymes; a TSH, as hyperthyroidism may precipitate CHF; and a BNP (B-type natriuretic peptide) secreted by the ventricles, which elevates in response to volume expansion and pressure overload. A chest X-ray should be preformed to evaluate for consolidation, pulmonary venous congestion, and cardiomegaly.

NOTES:

PATIENT NAME: TRACY HART
Clinical Setting: Family Practice Outpatient Office

A 15 y/o female presents with palpitations
Vital Signs
Blood pressure: 112/60
Pulse: 128 bpm regular
Respirations: 12 per minute
Temperature: 99°F
Weight: 110 lbs
Height: 5'8"
Pain: 0 out of 10

PATIENT NAME: TRACY HART
Clinical Setting: Family Practice Outpatient Office

Subjective

Objective

Assessment

Plan

CC: A 15 y/o female presents with palpitations

History			Performed
	1	Introduces self.	
	2	Explains role of provider.	
	3	Opening question: What brings you in today?	My heart's been racing.
Chronology/	4	When did you **first notice it**?	A couple of weeks ago.
Onset	5	What were you **doing when it occurred**?	Maybe riding bikes.
	6	Have you ever had this **before**?	I don't think so.
	7	Does it come on **suddenly or gradually**?	I'd say gradually.
Description/	8	Is it **constant** or does it **come and go**?	It's constant.
Duration	9	How **fast** does it go?	It's over a hundred.
Exacerbation	10	Does anything make it **worse**?	Not really.
Remission	11	Does anything make it **better**?	It gets faster when I'm really active.
Symptoms	12	Do you have any **stress or anxiety**?	Not really.
associated	13	Do you feel **nervous**?	Yes.
	14	Any **chest pain**?	No.
	15	**Shortness of breath**?	No.
	16	**Fever or chills**?	No.
	17	**Nausea or vomiting**?	No.
	18	**Weight loss or gain**?	Yes, I've lost 20 pounds in 3 months.
	19	Are you frequently **hungry or thirsty**?	Mom says I eat like a horse.
	20	Have you ever **caused yourself to vomit**?	No way.
	21	**Heat or cold intolerance**?	I'm never cold.
	22	**Diarrhea or constipation**?	Not really.
	23	Do you **pee frequently**?	No.
Medical Hx	24	Do you have any other **medical conditions**?	No.
Medications	25	Are you on any **medications**?	No.
	26	Do you take any **over the counter** medications?	Tylenol with my periods.
Allergies	27	Do you have any allergies?	No.
Social Hx	28	Individually: Do you **smoke, drink, or do drugs**?	No.
Sexual Hx	29	**First day last normal menstrual period**?	About 3 weeks ago.

Performed

	30	Has there been any **change to your periods**?		They only last about 2 days now. They use to last 5.
	31	Are you **sexually active**?		No way!

Physical Examination

	32	Informs patient that the physical exam is to begin.		
	33	Washes hands for 15 seconds.		
Vitals	34	Correctly performs vitals if appropriate.		Repeat pulse 120
General	35	Assess for **distress, tremors**		Tremors of hands
Skin	36	Assess for hair and **skin texture, and hair loss**		Warm, smooth, moist skin
	37	Assess for **excoriations of the fingers**		None
HEENT	38	Assess for **exophthalmia**		None
	39	Assess for **dental erosions**		None
Neck	40	Inspection	**Symmetry and masses**	Symmetrical, mild thyroidmegaly
	41	Palpation	**Masses and thyroidmegaly**	Thyroidmegaly without nodules
	42	Auscultation	**Thyroid bruit**	No bruit
Lungs	43	Auscultation	Instruct patient to **breathe deeply through the mouth**	
	44		**Complete inspiration and expiration**	CTA
Heart	45	Inspection	Identify **heaves**	No heaves
	46	Palpation	Identify the **PMI and thrills**	PMI 5th ICS 4 cm LSB. No thrills.
	47	Auscultation: aortic, pulmonic, tricuspid, and mitral		Tachycardia with regular rhythm. Accentuated S1.
	48		Identify S1, S2, S3, S4, murmurs, gallops.	
Abdomen	49	Inspection	**Contour**	Scaphoid
	50	Palpation	**Masses**	No masses
Assessment/	51	Give three things in the differential diagnosis including hyperthyroidism.		
Plan	52	Explained plan: lab analysis, beta-blocker if diagnosis confirmed, endocrine consult.		
	53	Asks the patient if she has any questions.		
	54	Thanks the patient. Displayed professionalism and empathy throughout the interview.		

Case Review #22

This is a 15-year-old female that presents to your office complaining of palpitations. Your initial differential diagnosis should include supraventricular tachycardia, anemia, panic attack, and hyperthyroidism.

The patient admits to a 20 lb weight loss over the past 3 months but she has not been dieting. An eating disorder (bulimia) or diabetes should also be added to your differential. Additional specific questioning should include self-induced vomiting after eating and quantifying what the patient standardly has at each meal. Symptoms associated with diabetes may show an actual increase in hunger and polyuria.

The patient admits to tachycardia, heat intolerance, increased appetite, weight loss, and a change in her menstrual cycles, which are all findings in hyperthyroidism.

She denies symptoms associate with panic attacks and states that she has not been vomiting.

The physical exam findings confirm that the patient is tachycardic and that she has a tremor in her hands. The patient has warm, smooth skin and thyroid enlargement. Exophthalmus is not present.

The patient does not have excoriations of the fingers, which may be present when a patient sticks their fingers down their throat to induce vomiting. There are no dental erosions present which may be a result of exposure to high acid level in vomitus.

In order to confirm the diagnosis of hyperthyroidism, a thyroid panel should be ordered. Once the results of the thyroid panel are received and hyperthyroidism is confirmed, the patient can be placed on beta-blockers to control the tachycardia until she is seen by an endocrinologist.

NOTES:

PATIENT NAME: BILLY ACHE
Clinical Setting: Primary Care Office

A 49 y/o male complaining of abdominal pain
Vital Signs
Blood pressure: 152/92
Respirations: 16 per minute
Pulse: 92 bpm
Temperature: 100.1°F
Weight: 168 lbs
Height: 5'9"
Pain: 8 out of 10

PATIENT NAME: BILLY ACHE
Clinical Setting: Primary Care Office

Subjective

Objective

Assessment

Plan

CC: A 49 y/o Caucasian male presents c/o abdominal pain

History			Performed
	1	Introduces self.	
	2	Explains role of provider.	
	3	What brings you in today?	I have a pain in my stomach.
Chronology/	4	When did it **start**?	A couple of days ago.
Onset	5	Did you ever have this **before**?	Yes, on and off for a few months.
	6	What have you **done for it in the past**?	I just take antacids.
	7	**When** does it happen?	It seems like an hour after I eat.
Description/	8	What does it **feel like**?	A gnawing, burn.
Duration	9	Is the duration **continuous** or does it **come and go**?	Continuous.
	10	**Where** is the pain?	Right here (*points to epigastria*).
	11	Does it **radiate** anywhere?	Not really.
Intensity	12	**Intensity** on a scale of 1 to 10?	An 8.
Exacerbation	13	What makes it **worse**?	Eating
Remission	14	What makes it **better**?	Antacids help a little.
Symptoms	15	Do you have any **heartburn**?	That's what I think it is.
associated	16	**Nausea or vomiting**?	I vomited once.
	17	What did you vomit?	Like this green black stuff.
	18	**Diarrhea, constipation, or dark stools**?	Yes, they're pretty black.
	19	**Fever or chills**?	No.
Medical Hx	20	Do you have any other **medical conditions**?	No.
Medications	21	Are you on any **medications**?	No.
Allergies	22	Do you have any **allergies**?	No.
Social Hx	23	Do you **smoke**?	Yes, a half a pack a day.
	24	Do you drink **alcohol**?	Yes, 3–4 shots and a beer a day.
Hosp/Surg Hx	25	Have you had any **hospitalizations or surgeries**?	No.

Physical Exam

	26	Informs patient that the physical exam is to begin.	
	27	Washes hands for 15 seconds.	
General	28	Assess for **distress and position of comfort**.	Patient holding epigastria.

Performed

Vitals	29	Properly performs repeat vitals if appropriate.	150/90
HEENT	30	Inspection Eyes	No icterus, conjunctive pale.
Lungs	31	Auscultation Instruct patient to **breathe in deeply**	Faint crackles in RLL otherwise clear to auscultation
	32	**Complete inspiration and expiration**	
Heart	33	Auscultation: aortic, pulmonic, tricuspid, and mitral	Regular rhythm without murmur
Abdomen	34	Inspection **Contour**	Moderately obese
	35	Auscultation **Prior to palpation, four quadrants**	Hyperactive bowel sounds
	36	Palpation Watch the patients face during palp	Patient grimaces w/palpation of epigastria. No masses.
	37	**Light and deep identifying tenderness.**	
	38	Percussion **Gas pattern**	Tympanic in the left upper quad
	39	Special tests **Rebound, Rigidity, Guarding**	Guarding of the epigastria.
	40	**Murphy exam**	Negative
Rectal	41	**Hemoccult**	Positive
Assessment/	42	Give three things in the differential diagnosis including peptic ulcer disease.	
Plan	43	Explained the likely diagnosis to the patient.	
	44	Explained plan: CBC, amylase, lipase, trial of H2 blocker, possible EGD.	
	45	Asks the patient if he has any questions or suggestions.	
	46	Thanks the patient. Displayed professionalism and empathy throughout the interview.	

Case Review #23

This is a 49-year-old male who presents with abdominal pain. Base your initial differential diagnosis on anatomy and include appendicitis, PUD, gastroenteritis, pancreatitis, and cholelithiasis.

The patient states that he has had this pain for a couple days and has been experiencing similar episodes for the past several months. The pain is described as a gnawing, burning pain in the epigastric area that is partially relieved with antacids, elevating the GI system in the differential. Eating seems to aggravate the pain, with the worse pain occurring about an hour after eating, which could indicate ischemic mesentery, a vascular atherosclerotic disease of the intestinal arterial supply.

He has a positive history of tobacco and alcohol usage. The historical data points to PUD but pancreatitis is still a consideration due to the patient's alcohol intake. However, pancreatic pain often radiates to the back.

The patient has had one episode of green/black vomitus and admits to black stools, a finding that suggests that the patient will need to be assessed for GI bleeding.

The medication history is important because NSAID and glucocorticoid usage can be causative agents in PUD.

The patient's BP is elevated and should be repeated. It will further need to be reassessed after his pain is controlled.

Hypotension, pallor, and tachycardia are signs of acute or chronic blood loss. If you suspect a major GI bleed, the patient should be assessed for orthostatic changes.

The patient has hyperactive bowel sounds, pain, and guarding in the epigastric area. Stool guaiac is hemoccult positive.

The practitioner should explain the likely diagnosis of PUD to the patient and the evaluation should then be explained.

NOTES:

PATIENT NAME: LOVEY DAY
Clinical Setting: Outpatient Office

A 76 y/o female is brought into your office by her daughter for forgetfulness

Vital Signs

Blood pressure: 152/68

Respirations: 12 per minute

Pulse: 72 bpm

Temperature: 97.4°F

Weight: 112 lbs

Height: 5'2"

Pain: 0 out of 10

PATIENT NAME: LOVEY DAY
Clinical Setting: Outpatient Office

Subjective

Objective

Assessment

Plan

CC: A 76 y/o female is brought into your office by her daughter for forgetfulness

(The patient's daughter answers the majority of the questions. The mother's answers are in bold.)

History

			Performed
	1	Introduces self.	
	2	Explains role of provider.	
	3	Opening question: What brings you in today?	**My daughter.** (Daughter answers, "Mom's getting forgetful.")
Chronology/ Onset	4	When did this **start**?	It's been going on quite a while.
	5	How has it **changed**?	It's getting worse.
	6	Did you ever have this **before**?	**Oh, I've always been forgetful.**
Description	7	**Describe** or give an **example** of the forgetfulness.	She can never find things.
Exacerbations	8	Does anything make this **worse**?	Not that I've noticed.
Remissions	9	Does anything make this **better**?	She seems better in the mornings.
Symptoms associated	10	**Slurred speech, facial droop?**	She can't find the right words.
	11	**Numbness/tingling/weakness?**	No.
	12	Have you **fallen** or **hurt** yourself?	**No.**
	13	**Anxiety?**	Yes, she's so restless.
	14	**Depression?**	She seems down all the time.
	15	How are you **sleeping**?	She's up a lot throughout the night.
	16	How's your **appetite**?	We have to remind her to eat.
Medical Hx	17	Do you have any other **medical conditions**?	**I've really got the arthritis.**
Medications	18	What **medications** are you on?	She takes arthritis medicine.
	19	Any **new medications**?	No.
Allergies	20	Do you have any **allergies**?	No.
Social Hx	21	Do you **smoke**?	No.
	22	Do you drink **alcohol**?	No.
Surg/Hosp Hx	23	Have you had any **surgeries** or **hospitalizations**?	No.
Family Hx	24	Anyone in the **family with the same thing**?	Her mother was really bad. **(She is not!)**

Physical Exam

	25	Informs patient that the physical exam is to begin.
	26	Washes hands for 15 seconds.

Performed

Vitals	27	Performs repeat vitals if appropriate.	BP 150/68
General	28	General assessment	Alert, no apparent distress
Neurological	29	Cranial nerves: performs II-XII assessment	PERRLA, EOMI
	30		No facial droop, ptosis
	31		Uvula midline, equal rise w/ "Ahh"
	32		Tongue midline when stuck out
	33		Shrugs shoulders equally
	34	Muscle strength: B/l upper and lower extremities	Equal
	35	Sensation: Sharp/dull b/l upper/ lower extremities	Equal
	36	Reflexes: B/l upper and lower extremities	Decreased -1/4 right arm and leg
	37	Babinski sign	Up going right, down going left
	38	Cerebellar function: Romberg, Finger/nose, RAM	Intact
Neck	39	Auscultation for bruits	Left carotid bruit
Cardiac	40	Auscultation: aortic, pulmonic, tricuspid, and mitral	Regular rate and rhythm
Respiratory	41	Auscultation: symmetrical approach.	Clear to auscultation
Mental Status	42	Perform a Mental Status Examination	Indicates dementia
Assessment	43	Explained differential diagnosis including Alzheimer's dementia.	
Plan	44	Explained likely etiology and prognosis: Unknown cause, progressive disorder.	
	45	Explained plan: CT scan of brain, Labs: CBC, chem, TSH, folic acid, B_{12}, VDRL.	
	46	Asks the patient and family if they have any questions.	
	47	Thanks the patient. Displayed professionalism and empathy.	

Case Review #24

This is a 76-year-old female brought to the office by her daughter for forgetfulness. You initial differential diagnosis should include Alzheimer's disease, stroke, cancer, infection, depression, and metabolic disturbance.

It is common for a patient to be brought in by a family member for memory impairment.

There is no definite test available to diagnose Alzheimer's disease. The diagnosis is made through historical data, physical and neurological examinations, and the use of diagnostic criteria.

Medication history should be reviewed for drugs that can cause mental status changes.

The patient's BP is 152/68 and 150/68 when repeated. Systolic HTN is a significant risk factor for stroke. A diagnosis of HTN should not be made on the basis of one visit. This patient should be brought back to the office two more times over the next 2 weeks. If the patient is diagnosed with systolic HTN, she should be started on an antihypertensive medication.

On physical exam the patient has decreased reflexes in the right arm and leg, a left carotid bruit and an up going Babinski on the right. This patient has residual from a past stoke that may be a contributing factor in her forgetfulness.

The diagnosis of Alzheimer disease should be discussed with the patient and her daughter. Information regarding patient safety should be discussed, for example, if she leaves the stove on and then wanders.

The plan may include a CT scan of brain to rule out hydrocephalus and mass lesion, and laboratory tests to rule out infection and metabolic causes of mental status changes; CBC, Chem panel, THS, folic acid, B_{12}, VDRL.

Discussion regarding starting the patient on cholinesterase inhibitors, vitamin E, and medication for depression and anxiety should occur once the diagnosis is made.

NOTES:

PATIENT NAME: KOFIB LUDD
Clinical Setting: Primary Care Office

A 62 y/o Vietnamese male presents with a cough (daughter is translating)
Vital Signs
Blood pressure: 150/94
Respirations: 24 per minute
Pulse: 110 bpm
Temperature: 101.5°F
Weight: 126 lbs
Height: 5'2"
Pain: 3 out of 10 with cough

PATIENT NAME: KOFIB LUDD
Clinical Setting: Primary Care Office

Subjective

Objective

Assessment

Plan

CC: A 62 y/o Vietnamese male presents to the office with a cough (daughter is translating)

History			Performed
	1	Introduces self.	
	2	Explains role of provider.	
	3	Opening question: What brings you in today?	He has a cough.
Chronology/	4	When did it **start**?	He's had it for several weeks.
Onset	5	Was the onset **sudden** or **gradual**?	Gradual.
	6	Did you ever have this **before**?	No.
Description	7	**Describe** the cough.	He coughs all the time.
	8	Are you **bringing anything up**?	Not much, but there's blood streaks.
Exacerbations	9	Anything make it **worse**?	It can't get any worse.
Remittance	10	Anything make it **better**?	No.
Symptoms associated	11	Do you have any **shortness of breath**?	Just if he's coughing real hard.
	12	**Fever or chills**?	Yes, especially at night.
	13	**Chest pain**?	Yes, his right side hurts.
	14	When?	When he breathes deeply.
	15	**Night sweats**?	He wakes up completely soaked.
	16	**Weight loss**?	His pants are falling down.
	17	**Orthopnea/swelling** of the extremities?	No.
Medical Hx	18	Do you have any other **medical conditions**?	He has diabetes.
Medications	19	What **medications** are you on?	Nothing, he won't take his medications.
Allergies	20	Do you have any **allergies**?	No.
Social Hx	21	Do you **smoke**?	No.
	22	Any **recent travel**?	He came from Vietnam 6 months ago.
Surg/Hosp Hx	23	**Surgeries** or **hospitalizations**?	No.

Physical Examination

	24	Excuses self to retrieve protective device.	
	25	Informs patient that the physical exam is to begin.	
	26	Washes hands for 15 seconds.	

Performed

Vitals	27	Performed repeat vitals if appropriate.	BP 150/94
General	28	General assessment	Appears chronically ill and malnourished
Skin	29	Inspection for **cyanosis**	None
HEENT	30	Inspection: nasal/buccal mucosa and pharynx	No exudate or erythema
Neck	31	Inspection	No masses
	32	Palpation: **lymphadenopathy**, all regions.	L supraclavicular lymphadenopathy
Respiratory	33	Inspection	Symmetrical rise and fall
	34	Palpation	Nontender
	35	Percussion	Tympanic without dullness
	36	Auscultation: Instructs patient to take deep breaths through the mouth.	
	37	Through complete inspiration/expiration	Guards right side with deep inspiration.
	38	Symmetrical approach	Faint apical rales.
	39	Special tests: **egophony**	Negative
	40	**Tactile fremitus**	Negative for consolidation
Cardiac	41	Auscultation: aortic, pulmonic, tricuspid, and mitral	RR w/o murmur, rub, or gallop
Extremities	42	Inspection for **peripheral edema**	None
Assessment/	43	Explained differential diagnosis including tuberculosis.	
Plan	44	Explained the likely etiology of a bacterial infection.	
	45	Explained plan: chest radiograph, PPD placement, sputum cultures, antibiotics, referral to Infectious Disease and the Department of Health.	
	46	Asks the patient and family if they have any questions or suggestions.	
	47	Thanks the patient. Displayed professionalism and empathy throughout the interview.	

Case Review #25

This is a 62-year-old Vietnamese male who presents to the office with a cough. The face sheet also tells us that he is febrile, tachypneic, and tachycardic, which are good indications that an infectious process may be present.

The patient has had the cough for several weeks. When a cough is present, it should be determined if it is productive, and if so, the characteristics of the sputum. This patient has sputum that is blood streaked, which should immediately alert the provider to the possibility of an active case of tuberculosis, although other etiologies exist. Respiratory precautions should be taken including a TB mask and placing the patient in filtered room if one is available. He admits to shortness of breath that only occurs when the patient is coughing hard and he only has chest pain on deep inspiration, which suggests pleuritic pain. The patient has fever, chills, and night sweats.

The social history is very important in this case as he admits recent immigration to the United States from Vietnam 6 weeks ago. Cough, fever, chills, night sweats, scanty blood streaked sputum, his malnourished appearance and his recent migration to the United States should make you think of TB. Other high risk patients would include those in nursing homes and the homeless.

The patient's BP is elevated and he will eventually need further evaluation to determine if he has HTN; however, his more pressing need is the infectious process.

The patient appears chronically ill and malnourished, and is found to have left supraclavicular lymphadenopathy and faint apical rales. The chest exam of a patient with TB is often nonspecific and may not reflect the true extent of the disease.

The diagnosis of TB should be discussed with the patient and his daughter.

The treatment plan should be reviewed including a referral to Infectious Disease and notification to the Department of Health. He will require a chest X-ray, PPD placement with instructions on when the PPD should be read, sputum cultures for acid fast Bacillus stains and long-term antibiotics (Isoniazid + rifampin + ethambutol). All contacts should be tested while minimizing exposure to others during the evaluation.

NOTES:

ORDER WRITING

6

All patients who are admitted to the hospital, be it for surgery, a 23-hour observation, or a full admission, will require written orders. When you begin to write orders, it is important to use a memory aid that will help you cover each important aspect of the admission. Several mnemonics are in use, such as ABC DAVID, and ADCA VAN DIMLS. You may develop your own memory device, but in each case, the goal is to write comprehensive orders that provide for optimal care of your patient.

Below is a review of the mnemonic, ADCA VAN DIMLS. As with all orders, each must begin with the date and time.

Date

Time

A—Admit: This must include both the provider to whom the patient is assigned and the location to where the patient is going.

D—Diagnosis: This is the reason the patient is being admitted and must be a recognized billable diagnosis.

The admitting diagnosis can never be "rule out" (i.e., "rule out MI"). Instead, the diagnosis should be "chest pain." This can then be followed by, "rule out MI."

C—Condition: This is a general statement of the patient's condition.

There is no detailed explanation as to what categorizes a patient as being in "fair" verses "good" verses "poor" condition. It is more of a basic clinical impression. Typically, a person being admitted to the Intensive Care Unit (ICU) would likely be in at least a "guarded" condition. Not everyone in the ICU would be in "critical" condition.

A—Allergies: This category should list all environmental, food, and medication allergies.

This should include contact reactions such as latex allergies. The reaction that takes place should be listed for food and medication allergies. For example, many people say they are allergic to aspirin; however, the effect is actually stomach upset and, therefore, not a true allergy but an adverse reaction. Still, it should be listed as the medication should be avoided.

Others will have penicillin allergies but do not know the reaction, which should be listed as "unknown." Patients often will tell you that they were told never to take penicillin because something happened when they were a child. This may not be a true allergy and may not prevent you from using penicillin as a last measure, but the notation must be made.

V—Vitals: This is the frequency for which you require vitals to be taken.

Occasionally you will need frequent vitals. For instance, if someone is postoperative from an abdominal surgery, you may need vitals every 15 minutes for the first hour but then with reducing frequency. In this case, you would write, "Vitals q 15 minutes × 4, then q 30 minutes × 4, and then q 2 hour." This type of order set allows for decreasing frequency of the vitals as stability of the patient is assured. ICUs have automatic blood pressure, pulse, and oxygenation devices. Keep in mind the total care of the patient and the nursing staff. Do not write for vitals every 15 minutes and expect that to run throughout the night. In one 8-hour shift, your patient would be woken up 36 times, which is not really conducive to healing.

A—Activity: (It does not matter which "A" comes first, allergy or activity.) This order dictates the activity the patient is allowed to perform.

This ranges from complete bedrest, where the patient would be required to use a urinal and bedpan, to ambulating ad lib, meaning that the patient can perform any activity that is tolerated.

If the patient was admitted for dizziness, it would be wise to write "ambulate with assistance," meaning the patient must be assisted at all times when walking. He/she can still use the bathroom but must first ring for nursing assistance.

If you require the patient to walk, such as for strengthening so that the patient can gain enough strength for discharge, write "ambulate 60 feet tid," which means the patient will be made to walk at least 60 feet three times a day.

N—Nursing: This includes general nursing activities that you request for the patient.

An example is measuring daily weights or the amounts of fluids taken in and given out. This could also be where frequency of dressing changes is written.

D—Diet: This is where the patient's diet is specified.

This ranges from nothing per os ("NPO") where the patient cannot take anything by mouth, to "regular," where no restrictions occur. There are two components to ordering diets. The first is the mechanical consistency of the diet from clear liquid, which is composed only of clear liquids, broth without any bits of food, and clear gelatin. Full liquid would expand the diet to include milk, which curdles in the stomach. Soft would include bread but not toast, and foods such as mashed potatoes. A mechanical ground diet would be regular food ground up and is often used in patients with dysphagia. A diet with thickened liquids would have all liquids with an added thickener for aspiration disorders.

The second component of the diet would be the content of the food. Diabetics should be ordered American Diabetic Association (ADA) diets, which must also notate the total number of calories the patient may have a day, for example, "2000 calorie ADA diet." A cardiac diet will include low fat and low salt. Renal diets will have low proteins. Each institution will have different components to the diets and you should visit the nutritionist to familiarize yourself with what is available.

I—IVs: This order is for intravenous (IV) fluids.

If the patient simply has a saline lock in the vein for twice a day medication injections, you may write for "Saline lock—flush with 2 cc normal saline every shift" to keep the catheter from clotting. If you write for IV fluids, you must state which fluid you want and for what rate. If you do not write for a certain amount or duration of flow, the patient may get to much fluid. For instance, writing, "Normal saline 200 cc/h," means that the fluid will continue at 200 cc/h until you stop it. Currently, hospitals usually follow protocols where the IV must be written on a daily basis or they automatically expire; however, do not rely on this implied protocol. Instead, simply write, "Normal saline 200 cc/h × 24 h." This lessens the chance of inadvertently giving more fluid than you intended.

You must also write which type of fluid you want to give. For someone with a high potassium level due to renal failure, you would not want to give more potassium as an additive in the patient's IV fluid. Likewise, if someone presents with a low potassium level that is now corrected, don't forget to decrease the amount of supplementation or you risk hyperkalemia.

M—Medications: Note each medication with its name, dosage amount, route, and frequency to be given.

Review each medication the patient is on and ask if the patient needs it or doesn't need it. More than once patients have been admitted with high potassium levels, but as the outpatient medications were written for them, a potassium supplement was added to the inpatient orders. You are giving the patient with high potassium more of it!

Then review each of the conditions the patient was admitted for and be sure that you have addressed each one. If someone is admitted in congestive heart failure and is on 40 mg a day of outpatient diuretic, how have you achieved diuresis? This will not occur by continuing their current outpatient dose.

Be careful with abbreviations. "QD" is no longer used for daily dosing. Instead, write out the word "daily." Never write a milligram dose followed by a decimal zero (.0) such as "1.0 mg." If the decimal is missed, you just gave your patient ten times the dose you intended (10 mg). Likewise, always write a zero before a decimal if the dose is less than 1 mg, such as, "levothyroxine 0.15 mg." Without the zero decimal (0.), if the point was misplaced or missed, your patient could possibly receive 1.5 or 15 mg, which is 10 to 100 times the dose.

L—Laboratory Tests: These are laboratory tests that you want ordered.

You must delineate the specific labs and when they are to be done. If you write for "stat" labs, you should inform nursing or the phlebotomist that you need the labs drawn immediately. Writing a "now" order does not always constitute "emergency" in everyone's minds and may result in the labs being done sometime later that day. If you want labs at a specific time, they must be written that way. Labs can be ordered for daily blood draws or for one time only. If you want to limit the number of times for the lab to be done, you can specify that as, "cardiac profile q 8 hours × 2," where you will only get two more cardiac profiles done 8 hours apart and then not again unless new orders are placed.

S—Special: This section should prompt you to order things like imaging or consultations (as seen below).

A sample write up sheet is illustrated on the next two pages.

Date
Time

Admission Orders—ADCA VAN DIMLS

A-Admit to "where" and "whom":	1. Admit to General Medical Floor, Dr. Smith
D-Diagnosis:	2. Cerebral Vascular Accident, Ambulatory Dysfunction
C-Condition:	3. Stable
	Guarded
	Critical
A-Allergies:	4. None
	Medications
	Foods
	Environmental
V-Vitals (frequency):	5. Daily
	Q shift
	Q 2 h
	Q 15 min × 4, then q 1 h × 2, then q 4 h
	Q 4 h while awake
	Daily Is, Os, and weights
A-Activity:	6. Bedrest
	Bedrest with bedside commode
	Bedrest with bathroom privileges
	OOB to chair qid
	Ambulate with assist
	Ambulate 60 feet tid
	Ad lib
N-Nursing:	7. Neurochecks q 2 h
	Dressing changes
	Position changes
	Tracheal suctioning
D-Diet:	8. NPO
	Ice chips
	Sips and chips
	1500 cc fluid restriction
	Clear liquids
	Full liquids
	Mechanical soft
	Soft
	Regular
	Cardiac
	Calorie restricted
	ADA

I-IVs: ("what to run", "how much," and "over what period of time")

9. D5 ½ NS at 125 cc/h with 20 mEq KCl/L × 2 L

Product	Abbv.	Rate
Saline Lock		KVO
Dextrose:	D5	100 cc/h
½ Normal Saline:	½ NS	Over 2 hours
Normal Saline:	NS	
Water:	W	
Lactated Ringers:	LR	
Additives:		
Potassium:	K	
Bicarbonate:	NaHCO₃	
Blood Product Units:	2 Units PRBCs	

M-Medications:

10. Current Outpatient Medicines that you want to continue and New Inpatient Medications

Single dose:	Lasix 70 mg IV × 1 now
Daily:	ASA 325 mg PO daily
As needed:	APAP 650 mg PO q 4 h PRN
Limited duration:	Cipro 500 mg PO bid × 3 days

L-Labs:

11. | | |
|---|---|
| Stat: | CBC (complete blood count) |
| Time specific: | Cardiac Panel at 1300 and 2100 |
| That day: | CMP |
| In am: | Fasting Lipid profile |
| With next drawl: | Mg level with next blood draw Call with results. |

S-Special

12. | | |
|---|---|
| Imaging: | CT scan of the head stat CXR q am × 3 |
| Consults: | Consult Internal Medicine Eval and treat Social Work PT/OT |
| Specific dressings: | |
| Foley: | Foley to straight drain |
| NG tube: | NG tube to intermittent suction |

Legible signature

Errors should be corrected with a single line through the error followed by your initials, date, and time, for example:

~~D5NS at 500 cc/hr~~ MK 1/7/06 0635

DOCUMENTATION SAMPLES

APPENDIX A

Sample SOAP Note

DATE: July 20, 2006

TIME: 0700

CC (Chief Complaint): Nasal congestion and frontal HA × 5 days

S (Subjective): 19 y/o cf presents c/o nasal congestion with thick green rhinorrhea × 5 days. Also c/o b/l frontal HA × 3 days, increased with bending over, post nasal drainage, and cough with green sputum production especially in the am. Denies sore throat, fever, chills, SOB, and ear pain. Attempted relief with Sudafed and Afrin with minimal relief. No other medications. FDLNMP 10 days ago.

O (Objective): WDWN cf in no respiratory distress

    T—99.0 F   P—88   R—16   BP—110/60

    Skin—warm and dry w/o rash *warm well perfused*

    Head—frontal sinus tenderness to palp and percussion b/l

    Ears—TMs gray b/l with good light reflex

    Nose—mucosa edema and erythema with green exudates

Pharynx—minimal erythema, green PND. No tonsillar hypertrophy.

Neck—supple w/o lymphadenopathy

Lungs—CTA w/o wheezes, crackles

Heart—RRR w/o murmur

A/P (Assessment/Plan):

1) Sinusitis—Augmentin 875/125 mg PO bid × 14 days with food

    Disp # 28, No refills

    D/C Afrin

    OTC Ibuprofen 400 mg PO q 4–6 hours PRN

    Increase fluids

2) RTC PRN or with increased fever, no improvement or worsening.

_____

Legible signature

Format for the History and Physical

I. Date and Time

II. Identifying Service—Family Practice MSI

III. Source and Reliability—Patient and chart, poor historian

IV. History

    A. Chief Complaint

    B. History of Present Illness (CODIERS)

    C. Past Medical History (MMASSH)

        1. Medications

        2. Allergies

        3. Surgical History

        4. Social History

        5. Hospitalizations

    D. Family History

    E. Review of Systems

        1. General

        2. Skin

        3. Head

        4. Eyes

        5. Ears, nose, and throat

        6. Neck

        7. Breasts

        8. Respiratory

        9. Cardiac

        10. Gastrointestinal

        11. Genitourinary

        12. Peripheral Vascular

        13. Musculoskeletal

        14. Neurological

        15. Psychiatric

        16. Endocrine

        17. Hematological

        18. Immunologic

    V.   Physical Exam

        A. Vital Signs

        B. General appearance

        C. Skin

        D. HEENT

        E. Neck

        F. Chest

        G. Heart

        H. Breast

        I. Abdomen

        J. Genitalia

        K. Rectal

        L. Musculoskeletal

        M. Peripheral vascular

        N. Neurological

   VI. Lab/Test Results

  VII. Impression/Plan

Sample History and Physical

VISIT: 08/12/2005 1110 ER EMERGENCY CARE
HISTORY AND PHYSICAL OUTPATIENT (T)

CC: Progressive SOB

HPI: 84-year-old Caucasian MALE presents with progressive SOB × 1 month. Pt with Hx of Atrial fib and L femoral artery embolism one month ago with embolectomy at St. Vs, Coumadin since and is now in sinus rhythm. States he has been SOB since discharge. Admits 3 pillow orthopnea, DOE and PND without cough, fever, or chills. No sudden onset of DOE; however now gets sob after only a few feet. Denies peripheral edema. Records from outside hospitalization reviewed with no notation of an echocardiogram.

Outpatient Medications (including supplies):
1) ENALAPRIL MALEATE 10MG TAB TAKE ONE TABLET BY MOUTH EVERY DAY
2) NUTRITION SUPL ENSURE/VANILLA PWD TAKE 1/2 CUP ENSURE MIXED WITH 3/4 CUP WATER OR MILK BY MOUTH AND DRINK TWICE A DAY
3) WARFARIN (COUMADIN) NA 3MG TAB TAKE ONE-HALF TABLET BY MOUTH ON MONDAYS, FRIDAYS, AND TAKE ONE TABLET ON OTHER DAYS OF THE WEEK

Allergies: PENICILLIN—rash, SOB

PMHx: Leukemia, Lymphocytic,
　　　　Chronic Hyperlipidemia
　　　　Hypertension
　　　　Atrial Fibrillation
　　　　Cerebrovascular Accident
　　　　Anticoagulants
　　　　Limb ischemia

PS Hx: embolectomy 6/04
　　　　sinus surgery 1955

SoHx: Tobacco: d/c 1935
　　　　ETOH: 1 beer a day
　　　　Drugs: Never
　　　　Lives: with wife
　　　　Occupation: retire with Hx of occupational exposure to chemicals

Family Hx: Mother deceased at 76—MI
　　　　　　Father deceased at 52—unknown

Review of Systems: Denies the following unless marked positive
Constitutional: fever, chills, + weight loss, + fatigue
Integumentary/breast: rashes, lesions, hair loss, nail changes, dimpling
Eyes: change in vision, diplopia, eye pain
Ears, Nose, Mouth, and Throat: ear pain, vertigo, epistaxis, dysphagia
Cardiovascular: palpitations, chest pain, peripheral edema, claudication
Respiratory: + SOB, + DOE, + PND, + orthopnea, cough, sputum production, hemoptysis
Gastrointestinal: dyspepsia, nausea, vomiting, diarrhea, constipation
Genitourinary: dysuria, hematuria, urgency, hesitancy, frequency

Musculoskeletal: arthralgia, myalgia
Neurological: paresthesias, + weakness, slurred speech
Psychiatric: depression, anxiety, thoughts of hurting self or others
Endocrine: polyuria, polyphagia, polydipsia, heat or cold intolerances
Hematologic/lymphatic: easy bruising, edema, + fatigue
Allergic/immunologic: recurrent infections, triggers

Physical examination:
84-year-old WHITE MALE who appears the stated age
BP: 145/75, Pulse 59, Respirations 26, Pain 0, Temp 95.9°F [35.5°C], wt 163.9 lb
Skin: warm and dry, turgor intact. No suspicious lesions.
Head: normocephalic, atraumatic
Ears: w/o exudate, TMs gray b/l with good light reflex
Nose: w/o exudate
Eyes: PERRLA, EOMI without icterus, exudate, injection. No shallow anterior chamber.
Throat: mucosa moist, w/o lesions, erythema, exudate. Uvula midline.
Neck: w/o bruit, masses, thyroidmegaly, JVD
Lungs: Distant breath sounds with bibasilar crackle. w/o wheezes.
Heart: Reg rhythm w/o murmur but possible faint S3
Breast: No masses, discharge, dimpling, skin changes
Lymphatics: No cervical, axillary or inguinal lymphadenopathy
Abd: Non-distended, normoactive BS, nontender to palp, w/o HSM or masses. No rebound, rigidity or guarding. No pulsatile masses.
Ext: w/o clubbing, cyanosis, or edema
Neuro: Alert and oriented, CN II-XII intact. Reflexes 2/4 throughout.
Strength: 5/5 b/l upper and lower ext. No focal deficits. Downgoing Babinski b/l.
Rectal: w/o masses, prostate smooth w/o nodules, heme-negative.
Genital: Incontinent of Urine, testicles descended bilaterally without masses, nodules, tenderness. No hernias.

CXR: cardiomegaly
ECG: sinus with 1st degree block and Inf. q seen on prior ECG 6/04

Impression/Plan: Admit to medicine
1) Congestive heart failure with hypoxia on RA
    O2 supplementation, may need home O2
    Lasix 20 mg PO now and bid, on ACEI
    Measure Is and Os , daily weight
    Order echocardiogram
2) Leukemia, Lymphocytic, Chronic—improving WBC
3) HYPERTENSION—mild elevation, follow trends on ACEI
4) Atrial Fibrillation—now sinus
    Hx of femoral artery thrombosis, no acute ischemia
    Coumadin with therapeutic INR
5) Hx of cerebrovascular accident—no acute change

Kauffman, Mark K., DO

COMMON MEDICAL ABBREVIATIONS

APPENDIX B

AAA	Abdominal aortic aneurysm
A&O × 3	Alert and oriented to person, place, and time
Abd	Abdomen
LLQ	Left lower quadrant
LUQ	Left upper quadrant
RLQ	Right lower quadrant
RUQ	Right upper quadrant
ADL	Activities of daily living
AD	Auric dexter (right ear)
APAP	Acetaminophen
AS	Auric sinister (left ear)
ASA	Aspirin
AU	Both ears
AKA	Also known as
AKA	Above the knee amputation
AMI	Acute myocardial infarction
AP/lat	Anteroposterior and lateral views
AROM	Active range of motion
b/l	Bilateral
BKA	Below knee amputation
Bid	Twice a day
BPH	Benign prostatic hypertrophy
BRBPR	Bright red blood per rectum
BS	Breath sounds or bowel sounds
BSE	Breast self-examination
c/o	Complains of
C&S	Culture and sensitivity
CABG	Coronary artery bypass graft (×2, ×3, ×4, depending number of grafts)
CAD	Coronary artery disease
CHF	Congestive heart failure
CN II-XII	Cranial Nerves II through XII

COPD	Chronic obstructive pulmonary disease	HBP	High blood pressure
CTA	Clear to auscultation	HEENT	Head, eyes, ears, nose, and throat
CVA	Cerebrovascular accident	HJR	Hepatojugular reflux
CVA	Costal vertebral angle	H/O	History of
CXR	Chest X-ray	HPI	History of present illness
D/C	Discharge	HS	At night, bedtime
DC	Discontinued	HSM	Hepatosplenomegaly
DJD	Degenerative joint disease	HTN	Hypertension
DM	Diabetes mellitus	Hx	History
DNR	Do not resuscitate	IDDM	Insulin dependent diabetes mellitus (also called Type 1 or juvenile diabetes mellitus)
DOA	Dead on arrival		
DOB	Date of birth	Infx	Infection
DOE	Dyspnea on exertion	I&D	Incision and drainage
DTRs	Deep tendon reflexes	JVD	Jugular venous distention
DUB	Dysfunctional uterine bleeding	L	Left
Dx	Diagnosis	LLE	Left lower extremity
DVT	Deep vein thrombosis	LLL	Left lower lobe (of lung)
EAC	External auditory canal	LLQ	Left lower quadrant
EGD	Esophagogastroduodenoscopy	LUL	Left upper lobe (of lung)
ENT	Ear, nose, and throat	LUQ	Left upper quadrant
EOMI	Extra ocular movements intact	LMP	Last menstrual period
ETOH	Ethanol	LOC	Loss of consciousness
Ext	Extremity	LUE	Left upper extremity
FDLNMP	First day of last normal menstrual period	m/r/g	Murmur, rub, gallop
		MCL	Midclavicular line
FROM	Full range of motion	MGF	Maternal grandfather
FB	Foreign body	MGM	Maternal grandmother
FH (FHx)	Family history	MI	Myocardial infarction
F/U	Follow-up	MVA	Motor vehicle accident
FUO	Fever of unknown origin	NAD	No acute distress
GI	Gastrointestinal	NCAT	Normocephalic, atraumatic
GU	Genitourinary	NG	Nasogastric
GYN	Gynecology	NIDDM	Noninsulin-dependent diabetes mellitus (also called Type 2 or adult onset diabetes mellitus)
H/A	Headache		
H&P	History and physical		

NKA	No known allergies	RML	Right middle lobe (of lung)
NKDA	No known drug allergies	R/O	Rule out
NSR	Normal sinus rhythm	ROS	Review of systems
N/V	Nausea and vomiting	RUE	Right upper extremity
OM	Otitis media	RUL	Right upper lobe (of lung)
OD	Oculus dexter (right eye)	RUQ	Right upper quadrant
OS	Oculus sinister (left eye)	RRR	Regular rate and rhythm
OU	Oculi unitas (both eyes)	Rx	Prescription
OTC	Over-the-counter (medication)	Rxn	Reaction
PERRLA	Pupils equal, round and reactive to light and accommodation	SH, Soc Hx	Social history
		SLR	Straight leg raising
PGF	Paternal grandfather	SOAP note	Subjective, objective, assessment, and plan
PGM	Paternal grandmother		
PND	Paroxysmal nocturnal dyspnea	SOB	Short of breath
PRN	As needed	s/p	Status post
PROM	Passive range of motion	subQ	Subcutaneously
Q	Every	Sx	Symptom
QD	Every day	TID	Three times a day
	(for medical legal reasons, write out, "daily" instead)	TMs	Tympanic membranes
		TMJ	Temporomandibular joint
QH	Every hour	TPR	Temperature, pulse, and respirations
QID	Four times a day		
	(for medical legal reasons, write out, "four times a day" instead)	Tx	Treatment
		U/A	Urinalysis
QOD	Every other day	UGI	Upper gastrointestinal
	(for medical legal reasons, write out, "every other day" instead)	URI	Upper respiratory infection
		US	Ultrasound
R	Right	UTI	Urinary tract infection
RA	Rheumatoid Arthritis	VS	Vital signs
RA	Room air	WNL	Within normal limits
RLE	Right lower extremity	WNWD	Well-nourished, well-developed
RLL	Right lower lobe (of lung)		
RLQ	Right lower quadrant		

INDEX